Any Day
with Hair Is a
Good Hair Day

ANY DAY WITH HAIR IS A GOOD HAIR DAY

How to Get Through CANCER
and Get On with Your Life

(Trust Me, I've Been There)

Michelle Rapkin

CENTER STREET
New York   Boston   Nashville

Scripture on pages 78–79, 128–130, taken from the HOLY BIBLE, NEW INTERNATIONAL VERSION®. Copyright © 1973, 1978, 1984 International Bible Society. Used by permission of Zondervan. All rights reserved.

Scripture quotation on page 78 is from The Living Bible. The Living Bible was published by Tyndale House Publishers, Copyright © 1971 by Tyndale House Publishers, Wheaton, Illinois 60187. All rights reserved.

Scripture marked as "(CEV)" on page 78 is taken from the Contemporary English Version, Copyright © 1995 by American Bible Society. Used by permission.

"CancerCare's Ten Tips for Communicating with Your Children," on pages 101–103 reprinted with permission of CancerCare, Inc.

Cartoons on pages 20, 39, 104, 113 are from Not Now . . . I'm Having a No Hair Day (University of Minnesota Press, 1996), by Christine K. Clifford, and appear with permission.

"The Most Important Rules for Cancer Patients," on pages 26–27, used by permission, HealthCare Communications.

Grateful acknowledgment to Emily Hollenberg and the University of Michigan Comprehensive Cancer Center for permission to reprint "Eight Ways to Know Your Doctor Is an Oncologist" (page 95) and "Positive Things About Not Having Hair" (page 96).

Center Street
Hachette Book Group USA
237 Park Avenue
New York, NY 10017

Visit our Web site at www.centerstreet.com.

Center Street is a division of Hachette Book Group USA, Inc. The Center Street name and logo is a trademark of Hachette Book Group USA, Inc.

Printed in the United States of America
First Edition: October 2007
10 9 8 7 6 5 4 3 2 1

Library of Congress Cataloging-in-Publication Data
Rapkin, Michelle.
    Any day with hair is a good hair day : how to get through cancer and get on with your life (trust me, I've been there) / Michelle Rapkin.—1st ed.
        p. cm.
    Includes index.
    ISBN-13: 978-1-59995-705-0
    ISBN-10: 1-59995-705-1
    1. Cancer—Popular works. 2. Cancer—Psychological aspects—Popular works. 3. Cancer—Patients—Rehabilitation—Popular works. I. Title.

RC263.R34 2007
362.196'9940092—dc22   2007012538

This book is dedicated to
Robert Steinbarger, my present from God,
and Dr. David Berman, my angel and God's instrument,
and Dr. Avram Abramowitz, my other angel.

a word of thanks

This book couldn't have been written without the many individuals who shared their own tips, tools, and information about how they fought cancer, either as patients or as those who provided care and support to loved ones diagnosed with it. Their great generosity of spirit has made this book possible.

My deepest thanks to:

Abbie Wood, the inspiration for this book
Hannah Bekritsky
Rosemary Barr
Ilana Burgess
Lubina Browning
Marian Cymbala
Catherine Credeur

Janice DuPlessis
Mary Kay Douria
JoAnn Dre
Jayne Donnelly
Lee Evans
Margaret Frederick
Nancy Goldman
Gloria Glenn
Veronica Gold

a word of thanks

Connie Hahn

Dr. and Mrs. Samuel
   Hassenbusch III

Sandra Hawkins

Laura Hearn

Matthew H. Herynk

Kara Herynk

Rosemary Herron

Karen Hill

Linda Hixon

Laura Holder

Susara Joubert

Jackie Lyon

Marsha Maurer

Wendy McCoole

Meg Nelson

Carolann Peters

Audrey Puzzo

Bruce Robertson

Luis Rodreguez

Kathleen Sanders

Josie Sethi

Carol Showalter

Ruthie Stevens

Jane Van Ginkel

Eva Vega

Francesca Villarreal

Sylvia Wagner

Kim Waymer

Betsy Wilson

contents

Never Had It Before? * Your Mind: You're Not
Losing It—Chemobrain * Mind Games * Dealing
with Depression * Matters of the Spirit * Prayers
for Healing and Peace * Maintaining a Positive
Attitude without Feeling Like a Human Smiley
Face * Retail Therapy Beats Chemotherapy

Cancer is so limited . . .

It cannot cripple love,
It cannot shatter hope,
It cannot corrode faith,
It cannot eat away peace,
It cannot invade the soul,
It cannot reduce eternal life,
It cannot quench the spirit.

— *Author Unknown*

just diagnosed

Welcome to the club to which no one applies for membership. It has local chapters in every town and includes men and women, adults and children. There are no criteria for membership except lousy luck. I know you can't wait to cancel your membership and burn your carrying card. Neither could I.

You've Just Been Named CEO

When I first learned that I had cancer, I was sitting at my desk at work. It was the middle of a difficult day, and when I learned that Dr. Berman was calling I was pleased for the welcome diversion. I don't know why it didn't occur to me that it's not a good sign when your doctor calls *you*, but it was only when I heard the devastation in his sweet voice that I realized something was wrong. He told me that a routine test had yielded a troubling result and that I needed to go for more tests immediately. He'd already made the appointment.

Within an hour I was at the medical lab, sitting in a tiny stall wearing nothing but an ancient cotton gown that was too thin, too short, and had too many openings. I'd even had to remove my earrings. When I heard "Rapkin!" I scooted past several nurses, doctors, and lab technicians, trying to keep whatever wasn't already showing under wraps.

It wouldn't be long before I learned that a big part of having a serious illness is waiting: waiting until your name is called, waiting for a prescription, waiting for a medicine to take effect, waiting for your hair to fall out, waiting for it to grow back.

One of the first side effects of cancer treatment begins within minutes of being diagnosed—before surgery, radiation, or chemo. In an instant, we go from being adults who are successfully raising families, meeting obligations, and holding down demanding jobs to being half-naked bodies waiting for instructions. At the very time we need to feel that we have power and control over our lives, we feel utterly powerless. That feeling of powerlessness is the first side effect. And it's important to eradicate it as early as possible. Believe it or not, I have good news for you: you may feel powerless, but you have a lot more power than you think.

The minute you were diagnosed, you became acting president and CEO of a major health concern: yours. Now you need to hire the best staff possible. You must assemble the most qualified team of experts you can find and put together an organization that is most likely to ensure the success of your business: the business of getting well and getting back to normal. This is big business. The stakes are high, and no one has more to gain or lose than you do.

Getting angry and shutting down and withdrawing will only make things worse. The Porrath Foundation for Cancer Patient Advocacy has found that patients who are the most proactive and informed—in other words, those who become CEOs of their cancer—have the best results and quality of life.

> The minute you were diagnosed, you became acting president and CEO of a major health concern: yours.

The first thing to remember as chief executive officer is that you're the boss; your staff works for you. That means your physician works for you, as does your oncologist, surgeon, and everyone else involved in your pursuit of restored health. I'm not suggesting that you should be a difficult boss; far from it. Good bosses bring out the best in those who are on their team. And you'll never have a goal that's more important to achieve than you do now.

There may be times, however, when you think that perhaps you should hire a consultant for a second opinion or look into another course of treatment. This is no time to be a "pleaser." Bosses have to make tough choices, and those aren't always popular ones. You will have to make some difficult decisions; after all, the buck really does stop with you.

Like any tough job, yours will teach you lessons that will serve you well long after this difficult time, which, by the way, *will* pass. One important lesson I learned during my cancer treatment is that *any day with hair is a good hair day*.

It occurred to me one day that all those times I'd stood in front of the mirror searching for every gray hair I could find (and pulling out a few), I'd been wasting time and feeling unnecessarily upset. Yes, gray hair meant I was growing older. So what? Growing older means that we're still alive—the very thing I was battling for with everything I had.

How many times had I wished my hair was a different color or texture, straighter or curlier, thicker or thinner, when just *having* hair is such a blessing? Have you ever stopped to think about what an incredible entity hair is? When it gets wet, it takes almost no time to dry. It keeps you warm without making you hot. When the rest of your body is sweating on a hot day at the beach, chances are your head isn't, even though it's covered with thousands of strands of hair. Hair replaces itself, unlike any garments we wear. And it keeps on growing for a whole lifetime; I could go on.

There was a time when I thought about these things every day. Six years have passed since I was diagnosed, and I don't think about them much anymore. But I pray that I'll be reminded—frequently—that when push comes to shove, most things that we encounter day to day, as Richard Carlson said, are "the small stuff." What's left, like a day with hair, is what makes our day a good one.

I lost my hair just before Christmas 2000. By that time, the chemo was beginning to take its toll in other ways besides making me bald. My energy was diminishing, my coloring was somewhere between green and gray, and, much to my shock and additional dismay, the chemo was causing me to gain weight. I was not a happy camper.

There were bright spots as well as disappointments. Frequently I'd open the front door and find a bag of homemade goodies dropped off by a neighbor. Several evenings every week for months and months, my friend Marie would ring our doorbell, holding a delicious dinner for me and my husband between two pot holders. I hardly ever had to cook.

One day, my son-in-law's mother, Abbie, called me.

She had recently battled cancer and knew all too well the challenges of going through treatment. As soon as I heard her voice, a new feeling came over me. For the first time since my diagnosis, I was talking with somebody who'd had cancer. It was like talking to a long-lost sister for the first time.

Abbie is one of the most practical, down-to-earth people I know, and shortly into our conversation it became clear that she had no time for self-pity or swapping sad stories. Instead, she said to me, "There are a few things you need to know that will help you a lot during your treatment. Your doctor and nurses won't tell you these things because they haven't experienced chemo, so they don't know. For example, make sure you always have tissues with you. Your nose is going to start running, and you're going to think that you're catching a cold or the flu. Don't worry; you're not. It isn't just the hair on your head that's gone. You'll be losing all your hair—including the hair in your nostrils. So there won't be anything to stop normal sinus drips."

What a relief that was. A nurse had already warned me about the danger of infections, and the thought of getting a cold or the flu was as frightening as the prospect of cancer had been before I actually got it. If it hadn't been for Abbie, I'd never have learned about "drippy nose syndrome," and I'd have worried needlessly about yet another lurking threat to my health.

Since then, whenever I meet people who have just been diagnosed and will be having chemo, I tell them to carry tissues and why. Invariably, they're so grateful you'd think I had just given them a big present.

In the pages that follow are hints, tips, information, and tools that hundreds of people have learned first-hand—many by trial-and-error efforts—to make life a little less stressful. They'll help you navigate your way back to good health.

First Things First

> Do what you can, with what you have, right
> where you are.
> —*Theodore Roosevelt*

When you're first diagnosed, there isn't actually a whole lot you can do. You're so busy going to doctors' appointments and taking medical tests that, for the most part, the only thing you have time to do is *wait*. However, there are some simple things you can do that will serve you well throughout your treatment and beyond.

1. *Get a notebook and designate it as your cancer notebook.* It's where you will write down *all* the information you need and things you might want to remember. Take the notebook with you everywhere; it will become a treasured possession. Buy yourself a pretty one—you'll be seeing a lot of it. The first things to write down are:

- Insurance information, including the insurer's toll-free number

- Telephone numbers and addresses of doctors, hospitals, labs, the pharmacy, and anyone else you'll be calling over the course of your treatment

- Medications you regularly take for other conditions (doctors will want to know about them)

- Questions you want to ask your doctor

2. *Make a cancer file.* Start keeping copies of all your medical records and test reports, which you'll have to ask for. You will need them when you get a second opinion. Even if you choose not to get a second opinion, you will need to keep complete files of your medical treatment from now on for everything from insurance claims to income tax deductions. Your doctor will charge a copying fee, as the physical records are legally his property.

3. *Keep notepads and pens at your bedside and around the house* so you can write down questions as they come to mind. Then enter them in your cancer notebook for your next appointment.

4. *Get a copy of your health insurance policy* from your and/or your spouse's human resources department. Find out exactly what is covered.

5. *Keep a log* of all conversations and correspondence with insurers, including dates, names, and outcomes.

6. *If possible, delegate the record keeping for your insurance claims to someone else.* This ongoing job is more demanding than it sounds. Unless you enjoy this sort of work, try not to do it yourself.

7. *Keep copies of every form* that you fill out and every document that you receive. Don't throw anything away.

8. *Keep a daily calendar* solely dedicated to recording all cancer-related events and expenses. Be sure to add things like wigs, prostheses, meals, transportation (including gas and parking), and lodging expenses. Many things will be tax deductible if they're not covered by insurance. Save all your receipts. The IRS can tell you exactly what is tax-deductible (www.irs.gov; 800-829-1040).

9. *File* all bills, receipts, and canceled checks.

Hurry Up and Wait

In the movies, when somebody is diagnosed with cancer, the medical team springs into action immediately; the patient is whisked off to the hospital, and the whirlwind of treatment begins so quickly that somebody usually has to bring a robe and slippers from home. The medical team is all on board from the get-go, and they work together like a well-oiled machine.

In the real world, on the other hand, things don't happen nearly that quickly. More often, the scene looks something like this. A test comes back to your doctor with abnormal (atypical) results, so he orders more tests. It may take a few days to schedule the tests, and then a few more days—maybe even a week—to get the results. Because there are often several types of a single kind of cancer (for example, there are more than twenty-five different types of breast cancer), it can take even more tests (and waiting) to pin down the exact diagnosis.

Many people, including me, say that this phase is one of the most difficult parts of their whole cancer experience. That may sound strange, but it's really true: *Not knowing* is one of the hardest places to be. Once we know *where we are*, we can start making decisions about *where we want to go* and *how we will get there*.

So try to take some comfort in knowing that right now you're accomplishing some of the hardest work you'll have to do during this entire process. And, ask your doctor how long it will take for all the results to come in and when you can expect to learn the final diagnosis. Typically it takes from one to two weeks. So much for the movies.

Breaking the News

Telling your loved ones, friends, and colleagues that you have cancer is one of the first difficult things you'll have to do. The Porrath Foundation for Cancer Patient Advocacy (www.porrathfoundation.org) offers helpful guidelines to help you break the news.

For example, when you tell your friends, prepare them a little by saying something like "Something important has come up that I need to tell you about. What's a good time for us to talk?" Be sure to find a time and place where you won't be interrupted. Go into as much or as little detail as you want. And don't feel that you need to keep a stiff upper lip or underplay the facts. Caretaker that I am, I often found myself trying to protect those I was telling from getting too upset by the news. What's wrong with that picture?

Remember, too, that there's no good time to deliver or receive bad news. The people who care about you want to be told sooner rather than later. Some friends of mine were very upset with me because they felt I hadn't told them soon enough. They wanted to be there for me from the start, helping me and praying for me.

Porrath also recommends that you write a script for breaking the news. You can prepare a friend by saying something like "I've been feeling under the weather lately so I went to see the doctor. The tests revealed a malignancy. So I'm exploring my options now."

Again, tell people as much or as little as you're comfortable with. The important thing is that you're allowing those who care about you to help sustain your body and spirit, just as marathoners need the support of those who stand along the sidelines, cheering them on or handing out water, to help them cross the finish line.

Choosing Your Oncologist

Once your diagnosis has been finalized, it will be time to choose an oncologist. This is where being CEO of your health really starts to come into play. You're embarking on one of the most important parts of your job: putting together your primary medical team. This consists of your primary physician, surgeon, oncologist, oncology nurse, radiation technician, and your oncology social worker.

It's absolutely crucial that you have complete confidence in the team you hire. They will help make your fight for survival a success. Your doctor will refer you to at least one oncologist. Make sure that you learn as much from the oncologist as you can. He will review your diagnosis, provide treatment options, and make a recommendation for your treatment. (Note: I refer to physicians as "he" throughout this book solely for the purpose of ease in reading. Obviously, there are many excellent female physicians.)

Choosing your oncologist is one of the most important decisions you'll ever make. Take enough time to make the best choice you possibly can. Don't let anyone hurry you unless you're told that time is of the essence. And most of the time, that isn't the case. The general consensus in the medical community is that in most cases it's well worth the time it will take for you to decide whom you'll hire.

We tend to assume that doctors possess all the qualities necessary to do a good job. In fact, the only thing their medical degrees indicate is that they're smart. That's a great start. But it's up to you, the CEO, to decide which of your candidates possess *all* the necessary requirements to do the job well. Those qualities include responsiveness to questions, no matter how many questions you have or how silly or trivial you may fear they are. This is cancer we're talking about, and your life is what's at stake.

The rule of thumb I recommend is to ask yourself one question: Does this oncologist treat you as well as you believe he'd treat his own spouse or child? If you suspect the answer is no, that's a good sign that this candidate isn't the one to hire.

Ask yourself one question: Does this oncologist treat you as well as you believe he'd treat his own spouse or child? If you suspect the answer is no, that's a good sign that this candidate isn't the one to hire.

You and your oncologist are going to have a long-term relationship—as in a lifetime. So you'd better be sure that you have confidence in him and feel some rapport. You're not looking for a friend, but you do need to have a sense that this person understands you, will take your questions and concerns seriously, and will take the time to make sure you understand what's going on. If you're interviewing an oncologist who obviously is pressed for time and makes you feel that you need to hurry up and leave, then do not hire that one. This is your first encounter; chances are you're both on your best behavior. If this is what you're getting now, trust me: it's not going to get better.

Get a second opinion. *Get a second opinion.* GET A SECOND OPINION. This cannot be stressed enough.

Why? For two critical reasons. First, you may have to choose from a variety of possible courses of treatment: chemo, radiation, surgery, hormone therapy, or perhaps a combination. A second opinion will either confirm the course of treatment that was first recommended or propose a different option. Second, you can compare the confidence/comfort levels you feel with each oncologist you're interviewing (usually this is called a "consultation," but "interview" is much more accurate). Remember, this relationship is going to last for the rest of your life. Even after you're in remission, you'll always have follow-up appointments with your oncologist.

Oncologists expect you to get a second opinion. Any job candidate knows that he or she isn't the only applicant being interviewed. One sign of a good oncologist is if he suggests that you get a second opinion. In fact, if he doesn't, chances are he's not the one for you. Besides, most insurance companies cover second opinions. You *know* it's a good idea if they're willing to pay for one!

It's generally agreed that with the exception of extremely rare cancers or those that are exceptionally difficult to treat, two opinions are enough for you to decide what course of treatment (or protocol) you should embark on. At a certain point, too many options may just make you unnecessarily confused or anxious. Plus, for most cancers, there are one or two widely followed protocols anyway.

But every person is different, and if you feel that you need another opinion, get it. It's your life—literally. Do whatever you need to be satisfied with the oncologist you hire.

TIPS FOR HIRING THE BEST ONCOLOGIST FOR YOU

- As you're collecting the names of oncologists to meet with, if you know people locally who've had cancer, find out if they recommend their oncologists. If you don't know anyone, ask friends and/or family if they know anyone you could contact. Unfortunately, these days, most people know someone who's had cancer. The reason for this, of course, is that there's no better source than a satisfied customer.

- Every oncologist who gives a second opinion will require all your test results, original slides, X-rays, and other paperwork. It can take a little while to get the slides (which you can't secure for yourself), so ask your doctor for them as soon as you've made your appointment for the consultation.

- Check references. Ask each oncologist you interview for a list of previous or current patients. Don't worry about offending the doctor—anyone worth his salt will respect your approach.

- Ask a friend whose instincts you trust to go along with you. That person can be an extra set of ears and can also take notes. You have a lot on your mind now and can use the backup. Perhaps most important, you can compare notes on your impressions of the oncologist.

- Be sure to bring your cancer notebook (the one in which you've written down all your questions) along to your interviews. Some people even tape their interviews, in case they're not able to read their notes or they forget an answer they thought they'd remember. The oncologist will be glad to let you tape your session, but you should ask permission as a courtesy.

As you're making your decision about whom you'll hire as your oncologist, remember:

- Be choosy.

- Be assertive. Don't try to change your personality. Assertive doesn't mean combative. The point is: just don't be intimidated. If there's *anything* you don't understand, ask. Remember, *you're the client.*

- Take your time (within reason) making your decision. Your doctor will tell you if time is of the essence.

- Make sure you're comfortable with the oncologist you choose, not only in terms of your treatment plan, but also in the way you relate to him. If he seems to be in a rush or unwilling to answer your questions in a way that you understand, he's probably not the one for you.

Clinical Trials

Clinical trials are medical research studies of new drugs or procedures using people as their subjects. They're usually recommended only if conventional treatments are known to have limited effect. If your doctor says that you're a candidate for clinical trials, he will help you look for the best one for you. The American Cancer Society Clinical Trials Matching Service, which is free and confidential, also helps find the most appropriate clinical trials for cancer patients (www. cancer.org, Clinical Trials; 800-303-5691).

QUESTIONS TO ASK POTENTIAL ONCOLOGISTS

Ask each oncologist you interview everything you want to know. Remember: you're interviewing this candidate for a big job. And you're paying him for his time. No question is too small. If there's anything you don't understand, don't move on until you do. Be sure to include the following:

- What tests do I need?

- How fast is my cancer growing? What stage is it? What phase?

- What are my options for treatment? What do you recommend and why?

- Will the treatments you recommend make me lose my hair? What side effects should I expect?

- Will I need additional therapy?

- Will I go through menopause as a result of my treatment?

- Will I be able to have children after my treatment?

- Will the treatment affect my sex life?

- Am I a candidate for clinical trials?

- What are the advantages and/or disadvantages of a clinical trial?

- Would you plan to stay in touch with my family doctor and other physicians involved in my care?

- Would I be able to contact you by e-mail? (Not many doctors agree to this, but it never hurts to ask.)

- Are there any particular problems that you would want me to call you about if they were to arise?

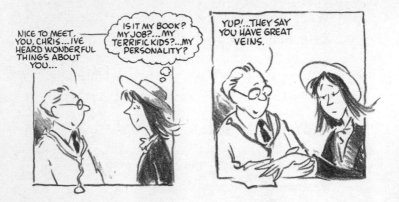

- How long do I have to make a decision on a course of treatment?

- What are the costs? Does my insurance cover the treatments you recommend?

- If I have chemo, what medications will be used? What does each one do?

- After I've completed treatment, can I expect the cancer to be completely gone?

After you've hired your oncologist, he will recommend an oncology surgeon if surgery is to be part of your treatment, and/or a radiation oncologist if radiation is to be part of your treatment.

QUESTIONS TO ASK YOUR SURGEON

- What kind of surgery will I have? How long does the surgery take?

- How long will I be in the hospital?

- Why am I having this operation? What are the chances of its success?

- What are the risks of this surgery?

- Is there any other way to treat my cancer?

- Exactly what will be done and/or removed in the operation?

- How long do I have to wait for the surgery results? Who will give them to me?

- What will happen if I choose not to have the operation?

- How long does it take for a full recovery? When can I return to work?

- What do the terms "clean margins," "lymph node involvement," and "pathology report" mean?

QUESTIONS TO ASK YOUR RADIATION
ONCOLOGIST

- What should I expect to feel during treatment? Will it hurt?

- How long is each treatment? How many treatments will I need?

- What are the side effects? Will I lose my hair? Will I get sick?

- What should I wear to treatment?

- Can someone be with me while I'm treated?

- Are there any activities I should avoid?

- What's the final goal of the radiation? Are you trying to shrink the tumor or eradicate it?

If You Have Breast Cancer (Not for Women Only)

We tend to think about breasts in connection with women, but men have breasts, too. Because breast cancer is diagnosed in women in far greater numbers than in men (in 2006, for example, there were 41,000 new breast cancer diagnoses in women and 460 diagnoses in men), we hear about its effects almost exclusively in terms of women. But if you or someone you love happens to be one of those men, the statistics don't really matter.

The risk of getting cancer increases with age in both genders, so as the population ages, there will be more cases of male breast cancer. A great many cases in men probably go undiagnosed every year precisely because we hardly ever hear or think about male breast cancer. When was the last time you saw an advertisement encouraging men to examine their breasts regularly for lumps or attend to breast irritation?

Men: if you notice or feel anything unusual in your nipple or breast area, go see your doctor. The odds are greatly in your favor that you won't have breast cancer, but you need to check it out. It won't go away just because you ignore it.

QUESTIONS TO ASK YOUR BREAST SURGEON

- What kind of breast cancer do I have?

- Has the cancer spread to any lymph nodes or organs?

- What treatments do you recommend and why?

- What are the risks?

- What side effects should I expect?

- Am I a good candidate for any clinical trials?

- What are the chances of recurrence?

- What are my options regarding breast reconstruction?

- Will I have normal sensation in my breasts after my treatment?

- How long is the recovery period?

- Will I need exercise and physical therapy? What kind? For how long?

- Is there a way to prevent lymphedema?

The Hire: Choosing the Best Candidate for the Job

After you've given yourself plenty of time to decide who the best candidate for the job is, make your decision—then don't look back. Don't second-guess yourself. You gathered as much information as possible, you've weighed the criteria, and you've made the best decision you could with the information you have. Of course, CEOs often hire consultants whom they have confidence in for major decisions, and so can you: perhaps it will be your spouse, or someone who has gone with you through the process. But in the final analysis, it's your decision.

> *Your medical team cannot read your mind!* If there's *anything* you think they should know, you need to tell them.

CONGRATULATIONS! You've just completed one of the hardest phases of the entire cancer experience.

1 You've made it through the excruciating time between that first telephone call and your final diagnosis.

2 You've hired the managing director of your medical team: your oncologist. This is the most important step that a CEO can take. I'm sure it doesn't sound as if these rank that high on the list of hard things you're being called upon to do, but take it from me: they are. Sure, there are more hurdles to come, and they won't be easy. But the difference is that you'll know precisely what your enemy, the cancer, is. And you'll know who is heading up the strategy of attack.

From now on, *you must REMEMBER that your medical team cannot read your mind!* If there's *anything* you think they should know, you need to tell them.

If something you're experiencing is causing you any anxiety, tell them. Also, ask about anything that you don't understand. Nothing is too insignificant. A great deal of the success of this entire endeavor depends on your keeping everyone informed. If you have to choose between telling them too much or telling them too little, opt for too much every time. This is one situation where there's no such thing as too much information.

The Most Important Rules for Cancer Patients

From *How Not to Be My Patient,* by Edward T. Cregan, M.D., Mayo Clinic cancer specialist

Know your diagnosis. Insist on seeing your X-rays, lab results, CT scans, mammograms, bone scans, and MRIs. Without knowing the details of your condition, you cannot access information about the problem on your own and make informed decisions.

Be in charge. Create an equal partnership between you and your primary care physician or specialist (oncologist).

Explore your treatment options. Get the big picture and then make your treatment decision.

Ask for a second opinion. Don't be shy.

Set up your support system and keep everybody thinking positively. Social connectedness is one of the biggest factors in explaining why some patients do better with serious illness than others. Families need to be supportive of the patient's decisions—no matter what those decisions are.

Do not second-guess your health care decisions. Don't look back. Plan ahead. Trust your instincts. *Carpe diem:* "Seize the day." Savor each opportunity. After all, today is really all that any of us has.

Life is a full-time job. Set priorities. Acknowledge your limitations. As a result of treatment, your energy, vitality, and focus may well diminish. It's up to you to decide what's most important and how to spend your time profitably. Time will take on new meaning. Make the most of it.

your body

What You Should Know *Before* You Start Treatment

- You should have your teeth cleaned and a complete dental checkup before you start treatment, and brush your teeth with a soft brush at least four times a day. Make sure your toothpaste has no abrasives. Both chemo and radiation are hard on your teeth and can increase your chances of getting gum infections as well as cavities. It's also a good idea to floss more frequently than usual.

- If you're terribly nervous before chemo or radiation sessions, feel free to ask for a sedative. Many treatment providers will be happy to give you one but probably won't think to offer it.

- Nausea is not "a given" during chemo anymore. New antinausea drugs all but obliterate nausea in

Keep Germs at Bay

To avoid infections, whenever you're in public places:

- Don't use other people's cell phones or public telephones. They're germ factories.

- Carry antibacterial gel with you everywhere and "wash" your hands frequently. Disinfecting wipes are great for surfaces (bathroom doorknobs, faucet handles, desks, computer keyboards).

- Carry a little bottle of homemade gargle instead of mouthwash. Mouthwash has alcohol and will dry out the tissue inside of your mouth, which has already been compromised. To make the gargle, add one teaspoon of baking soda and one teaspoon of salt per quart of water.

many instances. And if you do get nauseous in spite of a drug, it is very treatable, so ask your oncologist or oncology nurse if you can try a different one.

- Hospitals and cancer centers have social workers who can be extremely helpful. Even if you don't want counseling services, do ask to meet with a social worker. He or she can tell you what services you're entitled to and help you secure them.

- If you're going to have radiation, the technician will mark the exact spot (or spots) to be radiated with either a washable ink marker or a tattoo. Yes, a permanent tattoo. There are pros and cons to both: a tattoo will save you time, as you won't need to be measured and marked each time. And, of course, tattoos are very cool. Washable ink, on the other hand, comes off. Some people want to wear their tattoos as a badge of honor; others would rather forget the whole experience. Be sure to ask for what you want. If you don't, chances are you'll get the tattoo.

- Most chemotherapy treatments and some radiation protocols trigger early menopause. Before you start, ask your oncologist if you should expect this to happen to you. Consider a fertility clinic consultation if you think you may want to have children later on.

- Drink lots of water (sixteen or more ounces) before your chemo treatment sessions. It'll help flush the medication through your veins and will protect your veins, which chemo is very hard on.

- Bring a sweater to your treatment sessions; treatment rooms are often chilly.

- Chemotherapy sessions tend to last several hours. Ask your oncologist or oncology nurses how long yours will last. Then come prepared to be there for a while. You might just feel like resting, but you may want to read or listen to music.

- Bring a snack or juice.

- If you're on oral medications, it's very important to take them on time—but it's easy to forget to take them. Whenever you get your prescriptions refilled, sort your pills by dose, and then make labels with dosage instructions (save this information on the computer so you can print it out easily for each refill). Put the doses with the instructions in tiny ziplock plastic bags (they can be found in craft stores). Every day, carry the bags you need in your pocket. It'll make it a lot easier to remember to take everything on time.

- Don't hesitate to tell your oncology nurse or doctor if you think one of your medications (oral or intravenous) is making you feel particularly ill. If he can adjust the dose or try another drug that's just as effective, you may be spared unnecessary discomfort. Don't worry: your medical team will never give you "second best" medication in order to reduce your side effects.

MAKE FRIENDS WITH YOUR ONCOLOGY NURSE

Your oncology nurse can be an invaluable resource to you. In fact, she may be the most helpful person on a day-to-day basis on your entire medical team. For one thing, she's the one who will administer the chemo, monitor your blood cell levels, and generally know the details of your treatment better than anyone. She'll answer most of your questions about side effects and symptoms and can give you lots of helpful tips for coping with your treatment on a day-to-day basis. You're going to spend more time with her than with any other single member of your team. Oncology nurses tend to be extremely caring and capable; chances are you'll come to have great affection for her. It doesn't hurt, either, to bring her some candy or cookies, pretty sachets, or any token of your appreciation now and then. My motto is "Never underestimate the power of chocolate."

IF YOU'RE GOING TO HAVE SURGERY . . .

- At least one week before surgery, stop drinking tea or coffee, smoking, or ingesting anything that's at all addictive. You don't want to be recovering from surgery and in withdrawal at the same time!

- Get out of bed as soon as possible after your surgery; you'll save yourself a lot of pain over the rest of your recovery.

- Bring a sweater to the hospital; your room will probably be cold (I have no idea why—they always are).

- Your visitors may not realize that there are many others who are coming to see you. The result is that you, just out of surgery, will become host for several visitors each day. Don't let this become another burden. You're going to have to say something like "I appreciate your coming so much, but I think I need to take a nap now. Please come see me when I'm home again."

- Have a friend keep a list of visitors and gifts you receive at the hospital so you'll know whom to thank when you're feeling better.

SAVE YOUR ENERGY

You've now started your new full-time job, which includes spending lots of time and energy on going to doctors' appointments, chemo and radiation sessions, lab tests, and much more. Just traveling back and forth will be more time- and energy-consuming than you expect, so it's important to accept that you simply can't get as much as usual done for now. Once you accept that, you'll be less stressed and able to use your time more efficiently. Here are some additional ways in which you can use your time wisely.

- If you're slated to be treated at a hospital in another community, ask if you can get your treatment at a hospital close to home. Unless your protocol is highly unusual or part of a clinical trial, you'll probably be able to arrange it.

- This is the time to let your fingers do the walking. Get everything delivered that can be delivered, including prescriptions and groceries. If your pharmacy doesn't deliver, call around; chances are one will. Having your groceries delivered may cost a little more, but the energy you save will more than make up for it.

- If you have a top priority, then you automatically have a bottom priority. Prioritize. Make a list of every activity that doesn't need to be done, doesn't need to be done as often, or doesn't need to be done by you. Also, do the things that are most important in the morning, when you have the most energy.

- Remember that *people want to help you*. Often they simply don't know what to do. Delegate. You can make it much easier for them by telling them a couple of specific things that would be helpful to you, whether it's bringing meals or doing a load of laundry. Otherwise you'll get industrial quantities of lasagna when you could really use something else, like liquid hand soap.

TOP TEN WAYS TO SAVE PHYSICAL AND MENTAL ENERGY

1 Say yes whenever people ask if they can do something for you, because people want to help; it makes them feel more involved and useful.

2 Even if you can't think of something you need done for you, say, "I know there's something—I just can't think of it. Let me get back to you." If you say no too often, people will stop asking.

3 Keep running lists of everything: tasks that need to be done, questions for your oncologist, people who need to be thanked.

4 Keep pens, paper, and eyeglasses at strategic spots around the house such as the bathroom, the bedside table, the kitchen, or the den.

5 Put all the get-well cards and notes you receive in a single box or basket. Place a check mark on those that you've acknowledged.

6 Cut yourself some slack. Chances are your expectations of yourself are still based on your pre-cancer life. Since you have cancer now, it's time to let yourself off the hook for nearly everything except doing what you can to get well. Treat yourself as nicely as you would an acquaintance, and you may find you're better to yourself.

7 Pay bills electronically. You can do this online, or by telephone (call customer service and authorize an "electronic check" to be paid directly from your checking account). You won't need to write or mail any checks.

8 Shop over the Internet. It's safe and easy and even entertaining. All reputable sites are secure so that no information can be accessed by interlopers.

9 Designate a specific time to worry. When you find yourself worrying about something, write it down and save it for when your worrying is scheduled. You can give yourself a few minutes or an hour. Then you can get your worrying out of the way all at once.

10 Call ahead for appointments with doctors and labs and ask if they're running on schedule; if not, they'll probably be happy for you to come in later on in the day when they're ready to see you.

Hair Issues: Why You Shouldn't Buy a Wig for More Than $150

Losing my hair was one of the hardest things to deal with throughout my entire treatment experience. It took me a long time to realize that there were reasons for this apart from just being shallow, which is how I'd always judged others b.c. (before cancer). I began to learn that losing your hair is like watching a big line being drawn in the sand, separating your old life from your new one. It's usually the first visible sign of your illness to the outside world, and it's a shock to see yourself in the mirror or as you pass by a shop window.

If you're going to lose your hair (and not everyone does), your oncologist will tell you when to expect it to fall out, usually within ten to fourteen days. You can pretty much expect him to nail it within a day or so. It's a very good idea to shave your head at least two or three days before then. Trust me: you don't want to wake up one morning and find handfuls of hair on your pillow, or watch it all whoosh down the drain as you're shampooing it in the shower. It's even more distressing than having your head shaved.

- Ask a friend or loved one to be with you when you have your head shaved. There are wig salons and beauty shops that will do it for you in a private area. My husband shaved my head in the privacy of our bathroom. It didn't cost a thing, and you would have thought that Frédéric Fekkai had done it!

- There are very few good things about having no hair, but it will help if you try to look at your hair loss as visible evidence that the chemo is in your body and doing what it's supposed to do.

- Keep a lock of your hair so you can use it as a reference when you're buying a wig, unless you're experimenting with hot pink or Marilyn Monroe blonde. And even then you'll most likely want one that's your own color sooner or later.

- One woman made several small braids out of her hair, tied a ribbon at each end, and gave them to friends and loved ones with a note asking that they say a little prayer for her when they looked at them. After she went into remission, she hosted a tea for them. Ticket for admission: one braid.

- Almost immediately after you lose your hair (and in some cases, before), your scalp will become itchy and painful to the touch. That's caused by the treatment. Rub liquid vitamin E on your head to soothe and relieve the irritation.

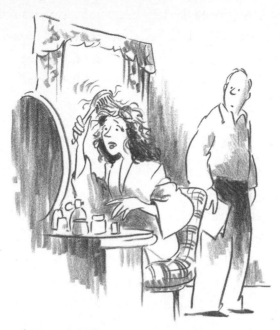

"TURN UP THE RADIO WILL YOU, SWEETHEART... LOUD ENOUGH
TO COVER THE SOUND OF MY HAIR FALLING OUT, ...PLEASE."

THE DREADED WIG

Getting a wig was very difficult for me. It brought home
the fact that I was going to be bald for many months. It
made me realize even more than I had before that I had
cancer; I hadn't imagined that was possible.

I decided to get the best wig I could possibly buy.
After all, it was going to be on my head eighteen hours
a day for the next several months. So I went to the best
wig salon I could find. They recommended that I get
one that was 100 percent human hair. The cost: $1,000.

39

"Maybe I don't need the *very* best. Do you have anything almost as good?" I asked. Yes, they told me, they had one made out of a combination of human and synthetic hair. It was only $700. I gulped and said, "I'll take it."

Some people decide that this is their chance to go blond or become a redhead or a brunette for the first time, but I went with my natural color—without the gray. I also chose my traditional chin-length style. I wanted to look as much the same as possible.

At first, I was so happy to have hair that I swore I'd wear it at all times, except when I was asleep. That resolution lasted about twenty minutes. Maybe I could have done it for a day or so, or a week, but this was a long-term proposition. So I opted for comfort and usually went au naturel when I was at home. I already had a new empathy for men with toupees.

Shortly after I started wearing my wig I began to pinpoint the physical discomfort I was feeling. My wig was heavier than my own hair. Heavy enough that I was aware of it all the time it was on my head. And it was hot. But there was another more uncomfortable sensation: my head was itchy. All the time. But what could I do? I assumed that was the price I had to pay in order to look like an earthling and I'd just bear it.

Which brings me to $150 wigs. One day I came across a wig store in a strip mall. It wasn't at all fancy. They didn't even have human hair wigs. But I was desperate.

My head had been hot and itchy for months, and I had months to go. I tried on a short synthetic wig. Oh, happy day! My head wasn't hot! It didn't itch nearly as much as it did with my "good" wig on, partly because the very knowledgeable saleswoman showed me a stocking cap, which provided immediate relief. So much for the top-notch care of a fancy wig salon. Nobody *there* had told me that. The cheaper wig also weighed far less, which also made it more comfortable.

On top of that, much to my shock, the synthetic wig looked at least as natural as my designer wig, possibly better. Even if that was just a mirage, I was definitely a lot happier and cooler. Whatever the cost, I was going to spring for it.

"How much?" I asked. "One hundred fifty dollars," the saleswoman answered. I couldn't believe my ears. "I'll take it," I said, before she could change her mind. I probably should have bought a couple more styles just for variety.

I put my expensive wig in the back of a drawer and never took it out. Granted, the $150 wig wasn't perfect. I still knew something foreign was on my head. But it was a godsend to me.

Hence my advice: *do not spend more than $150 on your wig*. It will probably be far better than an expensive one. Besides, if you decide you want to spring for a higher-quality one, you always can. If not, you won't have blown several hundred dollars on a wig that might well end up in the back of a drawer.

Of course, some people choose to go au naturel and avoid the hassle of wigs. I didn't do that, partially because I was working in a public place and felt uncomfortable being bald in that environment. Besides, in my case, bald is not beautiful.

TIPS FOR HANDLING HAIR LOSS

- Since you lose 30 percent of your body heat through your head, it's going to be cold when you go to bed. Cotton caps designed to wear to bed are often available at wig shops or from the American Cancer Society's "tlc" catalog. This is also a great place to get modestly priced wigs, wig accessories, and more tips about wearing your wig more easily and comfortably. You can also order a wig online (www.cancer.org) or through your local American Cancer Society office.

- If you lose all the hair on your head, then you'll most likely lose all your hair: arm, leg, underarm, eyebrows, eyelashes, and even pubic hair. And let's not forget the hair inside your nose! That's why you should carry tissues from now on, because your nose is going to start running—for months.

- Save your receipt for your wig! Ask your doctor for a prescription for a "cranial prosthesis" and your insurance may cover the cost. If it doesn't, the wig is tax deductible.

- Don't worry when your hair doesn't start growing back as soon as you expect it to; it takes a few weeks for it to grow from the hair follicles to the top of your scalp, where it becomes visible. Your hair will start growing back about one half inch per month.

- Use eyeliner and eyebrow pencil and brush to "replace" thin or missing lashes and brows. Take a close-up head shot photo before you lose your hair so you can use it as a guide for applying your eyebrow pencil.

- For a more realistic look when wearing your wig, lightly brush eyebrow pencil color along your "scalp line" before you put the wig on. It will enhance the illusion of roots under the hair.

SPEAKING OF HEAD WEAR . . .

The day came when I could no longer stand to wear a wig out all the time, especially when spring arrived. Scarves were a godsend.

- Be sure to buy eighteen- or twenty-four-inch square scarves. Larger ones are too big.

- The very best head wear I found was, I'm proud to say, something from the "necessity is the mother of invention" theory. I definitely had hair envy and bought every drugstore hairpiece I came across. One hot summer day I pulled out a ponytail and sewed it on the inside through that little hole in the back of my favorite baseball cap and *voilà* . . . the closest thing to my natural hair look that I'd had so far! I wore that cap well after Labor Day even if it was white. I highly recommend it.

- When your hair grows back, it may be different from your original color. My formerly brown hair was replaced with gray hair. "They gave me somebody else's hair!" I said to no one in particular. "It must be a mistake." On the other hand, a friend's hair grew in the exact shade of her former hair. If I were you, I'd assume the best, and if you do get gray hair, at least you'll have had several months expecting your normal color instead of worrying. Thank goodness for Clairol.

Coping with Side Effects

Fortunately for us, medical research has come up with anticancer drugs and treatments that have far fewer side effects than they did even a few years ago. Granted, there's still a long way to go, but people who are undergoing treatment today are actually fortunate that science has come such a long way. The list of side effects that follows is pretty comprehensive, and few people experience all of them, so don't get nervous when you read this section.

NAUSEA

Unfortunately, nausea is a common side effect of chemo. But there's good news: many powerful antinausea drugs have been developed in the last few years that can help relieve or even nearly eliminate it much of the time. Despite many months of chemo, I experienced extreme nausea only once.

Not only are there powerful new medications, but there are lots of different kinds. But no one formula works for everyone. So it might take a few tries to arrive at the combination of meds that works for you. Be sure to let your oncology nurse know how you're reacting. Then she can work on finding the right combination for you.

TIPS FOR COPING WITH NAUSEA

- If you find yourself frequently nauseous and confined to the bathroom for long periods of time, invest in a big, fluffy dog bed. One woman's husband came home with one for the bathroom, where he outfitted it with a pillow and throw. It didn't make his wife any less nauseous, but it was a lot more comfortable to lie on than the cold tile bathroom floor.

Invest in a big, fluffy dog bed.

- Eat a snack or a light meal before you have your treatment (chemo or radiation) to help prevent nausea.

- At the very first sign of nausea, take your antinausea medication. The longer you put it off, the harder it will be for it to take effect.

- Try to keep eating—something. Even just a cracker. It's important to get nutrition both to fuel your body and also to keep your body metabolizing your medications.

- Eat small amounts often during the day instead of having three larger meals.

- Eat bland carbs such as mashed potatoes, crackers, and pudding.

- Suck on Popsicles when you get bored with ice chips.

- Help stimulate your appetite by drinking a small glass of port or wine about half an hour before a meal.

- Don't drink anything with your meals; drink before or after meals.

- Drink ginger ale, ginger tea, or other ginger products—they help ease nausea.

- Eat very slowly (chew each mouthful thirty times before you swallow).

- Eat foods that are room temperature or cold.

- Call the doctor if your nausea and vomiting last for more than two days.

- Use scent-free products (deodorants, lotions) as much as possible to prevent odor-induced nausea.

FATIGUE

One very subtle but real side effect of radiation is what *doesn't* happen as a result of it. Because radiation doesn't cause complete hair loss, you probably don't "look sick."

Because you look well, people often forget that you're fighting for your life and don't have much energy to do a whole lot else. They don't mean to, but they often expect more from you than they would if you were bald or green. This is actually one of the worst things about fatigue: it's invisible.

There are other signs of fatigue along with feeling drained and listless, including difficulty in concentrating, talking, and making decisions, and being irritable. When you feel these, slow down and rest.

- Take several brief "power naps" or rest breaks a day instead of one long one. They'll actually promote healing as well as raise your energy level.

- Try to do activities that you enjoy, but shorten their length. That way you'll feel less deprived. Light exercise helps to relieve fatigue.

- Drink decaf beverages; surprisingly, too much caffeine depletes your energy.

- Rest whenever you need to. This is not the time to be "polite" or a hostess or responsible for entertainment. Don't feel guilty about telling those around you that you're going to rest. They can continue their visit among themselves.

- Eat protein. It helps rebuild muscle strength.

NOSE, MOUTH, AND THROAT IRRITATION

Many people who have chemo or radiation experience an inflammation inside the nose and throat. Here are some ways to soothe this condition:

- Keep your mouth clean and moist. Don't use mouthwashes, which usually have alcohol. Use baking soda or salt with warm water instead.

- Avoid acidic foods and juices (orange, tomato, and grapefruit).

SKIN IRRITATION

If you're having radiation, your skin will probably begin to look sunburned or even tanned where it's been radiated. You can expect it to become tender and possibly itchy. These are some ways to prevent or at least alleviate discomfort:

- Be sure to use deodorants that do not contain aluminum. Good ones include Tom's of Maine, unscented Dove, or natural crystal deodorants, which are easily found in any drugstore. A much cheaper and equally effective solution is to put pure cornstarch in an old spice shaker.

- Use lukewarm water and mild soap to wash and pat your skin dry.

- Don't use heating pads or ice packs on your skin.

- Don't use any skin lotions for at least two hours after your treatment.

- Don't expose your treated skin to the sun.

HAND-FOOT SYNDROME

Hand-foot syndrome is a skin reaction to some kinds of chemo, whose symptoms include reddish hands and feet, swelling, and burning or tingling sensations. To help relieve it:

- Use skin care creams such as Bag Balm or Lubriderm.

- Before you go to bed, apply cream to your hands and/or feet, and wear cotton gloves and cotton socks to bed. This will ensure that the cream is absorbed rather than rubbed off while you sleep.

- Use ice packs, gel ice packs, or even a bag of frozen vegetables to help relieve pain.

- Try taking a cool (not cold) bath.

- Don't wash dishes—hot water aggravates the skin.

- If you must wash dishes, don't wear rubber gloves; they'll act like a greenhouse on your skin. You'll just have to do without. Better yet, get someone else to do your dishes.

- Stay out of the sun as much as possible.

INSOMNIA

When you have laboriously accomplished your daily
task, go to sleep in Peace. God is awake.
—*Victor Hugo*

Another great irony of cancer is that just when you need your rest the most, insomnia often strikes, thanks to some of the fine ingredients in your treatment cocktail.

If you're taking steroids, they'll probably make you wake up in the night, full of the kind of antsy energy that makes you want to clean your house top to bottom. If that happens, go for it. Enjoy the energy, because the time will come when you wish you had it!

Chemo may well cause insomnia, too, but unlike that from steroids, you'll be awake and tired. I woke up in the early-morning hours almost daily during my chemo. Once I realized that I couldn't make myself go back to sleep, I started going into another room where I kept a blanket, pillow, crossword puzzles, many magazines, stationery, a radio, and a TV. Usually one of those things would get my attention, and then I'd go with the flow, not worrying about how long I was going to stay awake. Sometimes I'd get tired after ten minutes; other times it took two hours to get back to sleep.

Other people with insomnia have found these things helpful:

- Don't take naps during the day, no matter how tired you are.

- Use your bed for two things: sleep and sex. Find another place for all other activities.

- Don't go to bed until you're sleepy.

DISCOLORED FINGERNAILS AND/OR TOENAILS

I wish I could tell you why some treatments cause fingernails and toenails to darken and get ridges, but nobody seems to be able to tell me the reason. If it does happen to you, though, don't worry. It's yet another side effect. The experts tell you to keep your nails clean and dry, and not to wear fake nails. It's okay, though, to use nail polish.

DIMINISHED SEX DRIVE

This is a natural result of treatment. Don't worry; it'll come back.

FOR WOMEN ONLY: VAGINAL DRYNESS

Vaginal dryness occurs when menopause kicks in because of the discontinuation of estrogen production. Estrogen helps keep the vagina elastic and lubricated. Use water-based lubricants, such as K-Y Jelly, not oil-based lubricants, such as Vaseline, to ease the discomfort.

For Women Only: If You're Going to Have a Mastectomy

- Ask your oncologist for a referral to a plastic surgeon who is an expert in reconstructive surgery, particularly if you're considering having it at the same time as the mastectomy.

- Be as choosy deciding on a plastic surgeon as you were when you chose your oncologist. You're the CEO of your breasts, too.

- If you're considering reconstructive surgery, ask your surgeon about TRAM-flap reconstruction instead of an implant. Tissue is taken from the abdomen and moved underneath the breast area. The bonus (perhaps the only one in this whole ordeal) is a free tummy tuck. Another significant advantage over implants is that you'll have a more natural, faster recovery and far less follow-up will be needed.

- Don't feel that you need to make a decision regarding a reconstructive surgery right away. It can be performed at the same time as a mastectomy or afterward, so you can always decide to have one later.

- After surgery, when you drive, put a pillow between your body and the seat belt, it will protect tender areas and diminish any concerns you might have about driving.

- Move your arm around as soon as you can to avoid undue pain as your muscles heal.

- When being fitted with a prosthesis, don't buy an expensive medical bra right away. "Civilian" bras are often more comfortable and considerably cheaper. If you do buy one, make sure it doesn't have an underwire.

- Buy clothes that open from the front and are roomy.

- Use a small pillow to help protect a port-a-cath as you move around.

- Ask your doctor when you should begin to exercise, what exercises to do, and who can help you. Many women have had great success with the American

Cancer Society's "Reach to Recovery" program (800-227-2345), which offers one-on-one visits (in person or by phone) with trained volunteers who are breast cancer survivors.

Your Weight (Good News/Bad News)

Ask your doctor if you should expect weight loss or weight gain. In either case, it's best not to be surprised.

The Good News: If you've wished you could get those last few pounds off, a slimmer, trimmer you may well be in sight. Sixty percent of people in cancer treatment lose weight. Granted, there are far less extreme ways to reduce weight. But for me, the thought of *any* benefits from having this crummy disease was a ray of light. The prospect of losing weight wasn't just a ray; it was a three-hundred-watt bulb.

By the way, this definitely is not the time to *try* to lose weight if you're not gaining weight.

The Bad News: If you've wished and wished you could lose those last few pounds, hope that you aren't in the other 40 percent who maintain or gain weight during treatment. Much to my chagrin, I found myself in that 40 percent. I was devastated. As if losing all my hair wasn't bad enough, I was also watching the scale move in the wrong direction, and I'd had no idea that was even a possibility. I thought everybody who was in treatment lost weight. When I finally mentioned to my onocology nurse that I'd gained fifteen pounds (I'd wondered why he couldn't tell; everybody else could!), he casually assured me that "the chemo is causing that." I could have used that info a lot earlier!

Why do some people gain weight during treatment while others lose it? Some chemotherapies, medications (particularly steroids), hormone regimens, and the onset of treatment-induced menopause all trigger weight gain. In my case, the particular chemo I was being treated with was a factor. Apparently it had increased my appetite (believe it or not, I hadn't noticed), and since I'd expected to lose weight—and was also feeling sorry for myself—I ate whatever I pleased. Who knew that my new status of cancer patient hadn't made me immune to weight gain? To add insult to injury, since the chemo had thrown me into early menopause, my metabolism had plummeted. Needless to say, I was not amused.

According to the American Cancer Society, steroids in particular can cause extreme hunger and cravings. Knowing this in advance can help you curb your eating when you want to eat.

Water retention is also a common cause of weight gain, so reducing the amount of salt in your diet may help you keep the extra pounds off as well. It's a good idea to stay as active as possible and exercise regularly, as long as your doctor says it's okay. Even if you simply walk around the house, you're burning calories.

Managing Pain

> I've developed a new philosophy . . .
> I only dread one day at a time.
> —*Charles Schultz*

The best way to control pain is to get it treated early. The sooner you ask for help, the easier it will be to alleviate it. Don't hold off as long as you can without taking pain medicine. The only thing that suffering with pain achieves is that it forces your body to use your energy to fight pain instead of using it to fight cancer.

There are many safe, effective pain medications available today, and the more feedback you can give your doctor about what you're experiencing, the sooner you'll find relief.

The only thing that suffering with pain achieves is that it forces your body to use your energy to fight pain instead of using it to fight cancer.

As CEO, you need to bring up topics that those who work for you might forget to address. Don't wait for your doctor to ask whether you're experiencing pain. Tell him. Pain management is a very important part of cancer treatment, and experts say that, with the rarest exceptions, nobody with cancer should be in pain for long periods of time.

MOST IMPORTANT: Don't be a martyr! There are no prizes for suffering in silence.

Keep a pain journal. On a scale of one to ten (least to most pain), note how much or little pain you've experienced during a day. You can also track when and where pain occurs, how long it lasts, and the side effects you're experiencing from your pain medicine.

Nondrug treatments for pain include relaxation and breathing exercises, massage, biofeedback, imagery, acupuncture, distraction, skin stimulation, pressure, and vibration. The American Cancer Society offers extremely helpful instructions for things you can do yourself to deal with pain. See www.cancer.org (the section entitled "Pain Control: A Guide for People with Cancer and Their Families").

MOST IMPORTANT: Don't be a martyr! There are no prizes for suffering in silence.

Important Documents

All adults, regardless of their state of health, should take steps to let others know exactly what kind of medical treatment they want—or don't want—in case they're unable to communicate their own wishes due to an accident or illness. It's even more important for you to do this, not because you expect to die any time soon, but because it's the kind of thing that needs to be in place well before you need it.

According to the American Bar Association, even though every state has its own rules governing the documents below, health care providers generally will honor your wishes regardless of which form you use or where you drew it up. The ABA does recommend, though, that if you spend significant amounts of time in another state, you secure these documents there as well as at your primary residence.

The following are a list of documents you need in order to guarantee that your wishes will be followed if your ability to make decisions is ever compromised. They can all be rescinded or changed at any time.

APPOINTMENT OF HEALTH CARE PROXY/AGENT (ALSO KNOWN AS DURABLE POWER OF ATTORNEY)

This is a legal document through which you appoint someone who, in most states, must be at least eighteen years old, to make decisions about your care if you are unable to make them. That person has broad authority over your care and has access to all of your medical records. It is recommended that you name one person to serve at a time and that you choose at least one backup person.

LIVING WILL

This legal document allows you to specify your preferences regarding your treatment and care if you become terminally ill, or if it is not expected that you will recover from physical or mental disability or disease. The will can give general guidelines, such as requesting no life support if you are terminally ill. It can also include specific instructions regarding feeding-tube use or the use of a respirator or CPR, for example. A living will can be changed or canceled at any time. For more information, contact the U.S. Living Will Registry (www.uslivingwillregistry.com; 800-548-0455).

RELEASE OF MEDICAL INFORMATION

If you want anybody besides your first-degree relative to have access to any medical information concerning your condition, then it's imperative that you secure one of these releases for each person you want to keep in the loop. Like all of the documents listed here, this can be rescinded or changed at any time. But if you don't have it in place and you become unable to express your own wishes, then no exceptions will be made.

DURABLE POWER OF ATTORNEY

If you're not able to make medical decisions, this designates another person who can make those choices on your behalf.

Although it's a huge help to have any one of these documents prepared, it's generally recommended that you have all of them in place. Make sure to give a copy of each document to your spouse, lawyer, close friend, or physician.

your mind and spirit

Between stimulus and response there is a space. In
that space is our power to choose our response. In our
response lies our growth and our freedom.

—Victor E. Frankl

Remember: You Come First

This is the time to take care of your needs and put them
first—no matter whom else you're caring for. Besides, if
your own needs aren't being met, you can't take care of
others—whether or not you have cancer.

Right now, taking care of yourself means saying to visitors, "I really appreciate your visit. I'm a little tired now,
but please come back when I have a little more gusto."
Or, telling people what you really could use when they
ask what they can do for you.

Stiff upper lips aren't all they're cracked up to be. It's
okay to have a "sad day." It's okay to cry. Just don't get
too used to it.

How Do You Know How You're Coping with Cancer When You've Never Had It Before?

It only began to hit me that I really had cancer after the tornado of phone calls, diagnosis, appointments, arrangements, surgery, and everything else began to die down. Adrenaline is a wonderful thing. It puts us in high gear and turns us into temporary superheroes. But after the alarms and sirens fade, so does our adrenaline supply.

After the first days of crisis, I began to realize that I hadn't just spent two weeks starring in the limited engagement of *Michelle Gets Cancer* and was now back to my real life. Cancer *was* my real life. People would ask, "How are you coping?" and I realized I didn't know. I'd never done it before.

The American Cancer Society offers a series of "coping checkups" on its Web site for both those in treatment and caregivers. Apart from an overall "coping quiz," there are anxiety and depression checks. They are extremely short, easy to take, and, best of all, self-scoring. They can help you and your caregivers find out how you're doing (www.cancer.org, Coping with Physical and Emotional Changes).

It's okay to cry. Just don't get too used to it.

Your Mind: You're Not Losing It— Chemobrain

Not too long into my chemotherapy, I began to realize that my memory was fading fast. I was already worried sick about my poor body. Now I was getting worried about my mind, too.

At some point after the lapses started, it hit me that I was smack in the middle of chemo-induced menopause. Naturally, I assumed that my hot flashes, night sweats, volatile moods, and memory loss were the result of the menopause, and for the most part they were. But not entirely.

It wasn't until a year after I had finished my treatment that my sister called to tell me she'd read about something called "chemobrain." Chemobrain (slang for "cognitive deficits") is an unfortunate possible side effect of all cancer treatments, although not everyone experiences it. It isn't yet known why some people get it and others don't.

Chemobrain symptoms include:

- Short-term memory loss

- Difficulty concentrating/shortened attention span

- Difficulty retrieving words

- Difficulty organizing and planning

According to Dr. Christina A. Meyers at the University of Texas's M.D. Anderson Cancer Center, one of the best things you can do to reduce the severity of your symptoms is to introduce your brain to entirely new, different activities than it's used to. For example:

- Study a new language. If you've always wanted to learn Italian, now's the time. Audio courses and computer programs allow you to go at your own pace without leaving home.

- Play a musical instrument. If you never took lessons, get a recorder or a harmonica, which both are easy to learn. Or brush up on an instrument that you stopped playing long ago.

- Do crossword puzzles or sudoku.

- Learn to do needlepoint, or take a stab at knitting.

- Listen to do, different kinds of music and read different kinds of books than you usually do. If you're a mystery fan, read a biography. If you love Frank Sinatra, see if jazz strikes your fancy—or maybe you're a country music fan and you just don't know it!

- Try anything you haven't done before that will "surprise your brain"; it will be helpful.

- Listen to CDs that provide relaxation background music, guided meditation, and imaging.

- Ask your doctor if you're a candidate for Ritalin to help alleviate poor concentration as well as fatigue.

Chemobrain usually lasts up to a year after chemo ends, and it can last longer. No one knows what specifically causes it, but I for one am grateful just to know that my scary mental lapses were artificially induced, and I have a good chance of . . . What was I saying?

Mind Games

John Greenman

ACROSS

1 Whole ball of wax
6 Forty winks
9 Cries on cue
13 Rotund
14 Blown Away
15 Windy City airport
16 A day with hair
18 Sports event site

19 _____ de-France
    (region ringing Paris)
20 Show contempt
21 _____ on earth
22 Self-important ones
25 _____ capita
26 Cape _____ (Africa's
    westernmost point)

27 "Be prepared" is his motto
29 We all want to do it
30 Blushing
33 _____ group
36 Ornate
37 Jalopy
38 French star
39 It goes with hope and charity
40 Speedy sled
41 Dragged behind
42 Muddies the waters
43 Chorines
44 Unlatches, to poets
45 Teems
46 Zellweger and Adoree
47 City in Iran
48 Tom Sawyer's aunt
49 It's "the best policy"
50 _____ Paulo, Brazil
51 Feels remorse
52 Military cabal
53 Motorists' mishaps
55 _____ up the works (thwart)
56 Bridge triumphs
60 Light carriages

61 It's usually given in a parlor
63 Sticky stuff
64 Liquor, slangily
65 Winston Churchill said it
68 Kind of crust
69 Rathskeller quaffs
70 Cuts of pork
71 Molt
72 Alcove
73 Maternally related

DOWN

1 Hammers, wrenches, and saws
2 Bassoons' kin
3 Turner or Danson
4 _____ Wednesday
5 Pastures
6 U.S. consumer activist
7 Culture medium
8 Fork over
9 In the lead
10 The best things since sliced bread
11 Accurate
12 Match a poker bet

14 Hail; welcome

15 With excessiveness

16 Actress Scala

17 Computer data entered

21 Pinkish-yellow hue

23 Catches sight of

24 Rebuke

26 Air ducts

28 Argentite is one

29 Showers heavy sleet

31 Small seabird

32 Formal attire

33 First U.S. saint et al.

34 Idealized spot

35 Never underestimate it

36 Pixie

39 Diamond goofs

40 Hereditary

42 Parts in a play

43 Blokes

45 Gets sulky

46 Director Howard

48 Petition to God

49 You need it to get through cancer

52 Burlap fibers

54 Lolled; lounged

55 Judge's mallet

57 Celeb's representative

58 Mickey or Minnie

59 Drench

60 Next year's jr.

61 Give an account of

62 Make eyes at

64 City conveyance

65 Glasgow veto

66 Particle

67 By way of

Dealing with Depression

It's one thing to be sad. If you weren't sad about having cancer, that would be very strange. But there's a real difference between being sad and being depressed. At any given time, 10 percent of the American population suffers from depression. Thirty percent of cancer patients suffer from it; so if you think you might be depressed, the odds are that you are.

I've suffered from bouts of major depression in my life, and I can assure you that you really don't want to be in the middle of cancer and depression at the same time. One is bad enough, but in combination they're brutal.

ONGOING SYMPTOMS OF DEPRESSION

Symptoms of depression include:

- Exaggerated feelings of hopelessness, despair, worthlessness, and inadequacy

- Little, if any, interest in things that used to be pleasurable

- Crying often and easily

- Thoughts of suicide

- Loss of interest in sex

- Extreme feelings of worthlessness and guilt

If you experience some or all of these feelings much or most of the time, please, please tell your medical team as soon as you realize that they're not going away. Your body needs all of its energy to heal. Why force it to undergo the added stress of depression? Also, the medical community has determined that there is a strong connection between depression and a suppressed immune system, which is the last thing you need right now.

> The time will come when you wake up and realize that you haven't thought about having had cancer for one or two weeks or months!

Finally, don't worry about antidepressants. I know how hard it is to accept the fact that you might need them. But I can tell you from experience that taking them is like taking aspirin or allergy medicine. In fact, if you've ever taken Zyban to quit smoking, then you've already taken an antidepressant. Zyban is Wellbutrin, one of the most widely used antidepressants in the country.

Remember, don't suffer in silence. Don't just hope the depression will go away by itself. It won't. Tell your doctor as soon as you think that you might be depressed.

Like pain, the earlier depression is treated, the more quickly and easily it will be alleviated. Not to mention that you'll avoid unnecessary strain on your already overworked body. The time will come when you wake up and realize that you haven't thought about having had cancer for one or two weeks or months!

Ultimately it will not dominate your mind and your spirit. It will be a part of your experience, but not at the forefront; it will be a memory, but not a trauma.

Matters of the Spirit

Faith is taking the first step even when you don't see
the whole staircase.
—*Martin Luther King Jr.*

Whatever your beliefs are—or aren't—it's just as important to nourish your soul as it is to feed your body. For whatever reason, it's often when we're in crisis that we begin to explore things of the spirit, whether by prayer, meditation, listening to Bach or Mozart, or simply being quiet with our eyes closed.

The National Institute of Mental Health has even determined that people with cancer often have less anxiety, depression, and even pain when they feel strong spiritual connections.

Many studies have shown conclusively that prayerful consciousness has been shown to inhibit the growth of cancer cells, increase the supply of oxygen to the blood, protect red blood cells, and alter blood chemistry. Some studies have even shown that prayer on behalf of a sick person has some positive effect on the healing process.

Prayer has always been an important part of my life.

But after I was diagnosed, it became even more so. Not only did I find myself praying more intensely and mindfully than before, but I also wanted to be prayed *for*. In fact, when people wanted to know what they could do for me, I found myself asking them to pray—not only for me, but also for my husband and family and my medical team. That was the gift I wanted most. Trust me, I'm pretty materialistic, so no one was more surprised at this desire for prayer than me.

Most of the time, my own prayers consisted of my just talking to God (not out loud—the last thing I needed was to be given a second diagnosis: psychotic). Much of the time, I was pretty mad at him for letting this happen to me. I hadn't married until I was forty-five, and I'd been married for only two years. What if I didn't make it? So I'd rail at him. "*What* were you think-ing?" I'd ask. I figured that if God is God, then he can take my yelling at him. But I also asked for peace and strength and comfort—and healing, of course. During the process, I became less angry and more peaceful.

Prayers for Healing and Peace

Here are several prayers, for a variety of faiths, that you may find helpful. Each denomination is represented by a prayer that was written by a member of the clergy who is no stranger to cancer.

CATHOLIC

Peregrine, the Patron Saint of Cancer

Peregrine Laziosi was born in 1260 in Forli, Italy, to a very wealthy family. His youth was spent selfishly and was monopolized by material possessions. He found his way into politics and became very anti-Catholic. Peregrine converted, however, after beating Philip Benizi, a future saint, and seeing the holy man turn the cheek and pray for his attacker. Peregrine later joined the Servite order and spent many years in solitude. The gentle confessor fell victim to a horrific cancer of his foot that spread rapidly. While awaiting amputation, Peregrine spent the night before the operation in prayer and received a vision of Jesus healing his malady instantly. By the next morning, his foot was completely cured.

> **Prayer to St. Peregrine**
> *O great Peregrine,*
> *I am inspired by your faith, bravery and stamina.*
> *Pray that I can be as strong and prayerful as you were.*
> *Ask God to get me through this painful experience with*
> *   dignity and laughter.*
> *Pray for my supportive family and my loving friends, as*
> *   God sees me through to a total recovery.*
> *Amen.*
>
> *—from Saintly Advice*

PROTESTANT

*Eternal and loving God, in the midst of illness I will
praise your holy name.*

*Even as I fight this fateful disease, I will affirm that life is
good and a blessing to be savored.*

*By your grace, help me find something amazing to
cherish and thank you for daily, something, perhaps,
that I might not have noticed when I was well.*

*Firm me in my determination not to allow cancer to rob
me of my values or my personality, or alienate me
from those I love, including you, O Lord.*

Precious Father, get me through the hard days.

Hold my hand and do not let fear conquer me.

*Above all, open me to your healing power, for I pray to
you through your Son, Jesus Christ.*

Amen.

> —Rev. Dr. Noel Vanek, pastor,
> The Church-in-the-Gardens
> (Congregational), Forest Hills, New York

JEWISH

*May the One who blessed our Patriarchs Abraham,
Isaac and Jacob and our Matriarchs Sarah, Rebecca,
Rachel, and Leah bless me in my journey seeking a
Refuah Shleimah, a healing of Body and Spirit.*

Please bless my clinicians not only in treating my illness,

*but also in supporting me as a unique spirit created in
Your Image.*

*Please bless my family and friends as they support me.
May I be blessed to feel Your love through them. May
they be strengthened in Your love as well.*

*Please allow me to feel Your Presence in the mountains
and valleys—for I know that wherever I go, You shall
be there.*

*Help me to accept and love who I am in the moment—
emotionally, physically and spiritually—as I know
that You, my Creator who knew me in the womb,
accept and love me.*

May I be restored to a healing of soul and body.

    —Rabbi Nathan Goldberg,

      director of pastoral care and education,

      Beth Israel Medical Center ACPE supervisor,

      The HealthCare Chaplaincy, New York, New York

ISLAMIC

*With G-D's name the merciful benefactor, the merciful
Redeemer,*

*Dear G-D, please give us what is good in this life, and
what is good in the next life, and save us, because
nothing can save us except you.*

We humbly ask you to heal us, very soon.

*Please make this process easy for us and do not place a
burden on us greater than we can bear.*

We also ask that you bless our families, because we don't
know why we are tested with so much illness and
hardships in our lives.
Please give them the strength, the courage and the faith to
deal with anything that comes in the future.
Bless the doctors and nurses who care for us, that they
make right decisions.
Now we ask you to bless the sick and infirm, especially
the children, wherever they may be on this earth,
because after all the earth is our home.
Above all, please bless us to be well and continue to live
a long, good and healthy life, if it pleases you.
Amen.

—Imam Yusuf Hasan, B.C.C., The HealthCare
Chaplaincy, and assistant at Malcolm Shabazz
Masjid, New York, New York

ENCOURAGEMENT, COMFORT, AND STRENGTH FROM THE BIBLE

I read some books while I was in treatment that encouraged me and gave me new insights into the spiritual aspects of going through cancer, some specific to the disease and others more general. But the most encouraging, comforting ones for me that gave me injections of peace and strength were from the Bible. I've included some passages from a few of them here that were among the most helpful to me.

> But now the Lord who created you, O Israel, says: "Do not be afraid, for I have ransomed you; I have called you by name; you are mine. When you go through deep waters and great trouble, I will be with you. When you go through rivers of difficulty, you will not drown! When you walk through the fire of oppression, you will not be burned up—the flames will not consume you."
>
> — Isaiah 43:1–2, *The Living Bible*

> I look to the hills! Where will I find help? It will come from the LORD, who created the heavens and the earth.—Psalm 121:1–2, *CEV*

> Even though I walk through the valley of the shadow of death, I will fear no evil, for you are with me.—Psalm 23:4, *NIV*

> Do not fear, I will help you.—Isaiah 41:13, *NIV*

> The LORD bless you and keep you; the LORD make his face to shine upon you and be gracious to you; the LORD turn his face toward you and give you peace.—Numbers 6:24–26, *NIV*

Be strong and courageous. Do not be terrified; do not be discouraged, for the LORD your God will be with you wherever you go.—Joshua 1:9, *NIV*

He rescues and he saves; he performs signs and wonders in the heavens and on the earth. He has rescued Daniel from the power of the lions.

—Daniel 6:27, *NIV*

Maintaining a Positive Attitude without Feeling Like a Human Smiley Face

THE HOUSE OF A THOUSAND MIRRORS

Long ago in a tiny village, there was a place called the House of a Thousand Mirrors. A little dog decided to visit the house. He was an unhappy dog, and his natural expression was a cross between a scowl and a sneer. As he entered the large house, he saw a thousand mean- and scary-looking dogs staring back at him. He immediately backed away and let out a low growl to protect himself, and, just as he did, all one thousand of the mean dogs growled back at him. Of course he ran out of the house immediately and thought "What a terrible place that is. I'll never go back there again."

Not long afterward, another dog decided to visit the house. As he approached, he saw how beautiful and inviting it looked and couldn't wait to go inside. He smiled and wagged his tail in anticipation of his adventure. As he pushed open the door, he was greeted by a thousand dogs with wagging tails and big smiles approaching him. Of course he was thrilled; he had a thousand new friends he was sure would become his buddies.

The moral of this folktale, of course, is that the world gives back to us what we give out to the world. That's not to say we should pretend that everything's great when in fact we're going through one of the hardest challenges of our lives. But it *is* true that the more positive you can be right now, the more smiling puppies you'll have to cheer you on.

HELPFUL SELF-TALK

Often, in an effort to make you feel better, people will say some pretty annoying things; "infuriating" is probably a more accurate term. Having cancer is *not* a blessing in disguise. The fact that you don't have a worse cancer is not terribly comforting. As wonderful as it is to learn how many people love and care about you, there are other ways to learn that that aren't nearly as dangerous, devastating, or life-altering as having cancer.

But there are some things that are true and can bring comfort and a new perspective on this crummy situation. These are some that have been of help to me:

- *A year from today this will be behind me.*

- *A year from today, I'll have hair!*

- *My lack of hair means that the chemo is working.*

- *I am* not *a statistic.*

- *I am the CEO of my health.* I have control over many things, and this is the time for me to take hold of and maintain and use that power.

- *There are more people who care deeply and want to support me* now than perhaps at any time in my life. I need to accept their generosity, and one day I will reciprocate. If they sometimes say dumb things, it's because they're frightened on my behalf. I need to give them the benefit of the doubt and accept with grace their stabs at comforting me.

- *Cancer is not a death sentence.* In fact, more people die of heart disease every year than of cancer. Yet we don't view people with heart disease as living under the specter of death. Just because an idea is commonly believed, that doesn't make it true.

- *Just because your prognosis is better than mine doesn't mean you'll outlive me!* Granted, this is a little hard-nosed, and it's probably better if you don't go around saying it to people. But the truth is nobody knows what will happen next week, or tomorrow, or in an hour.

- *Cancer sucks.* There are pins, T-shirts, and baseball caps that say "CANCER SUCKS." It's short and to the point and, in my opinion, sums up the situation to a tee. For some mysterious reason, it made me feel better just to say those two little words every now and then.

- *I'm going to make cancer history.* (Get it? Make cancer history . . .)

- *Just because I'm not cured yet, it doesn't mean that I can't experience healing.* As you know, there isn't a lot about cancer that could be called "beneficial." But like many other hard experiences in life, even this terrible journey can be—in fact, often is—a catalyst for healing in areas that will serve us well both in the short run and the long run. Chances are you've already experienced an outpouring of care and kindness from others whom you wouldn't have expected to be so giving. Cancer causes us to reexamine our priorities and often triggers new, healthier decisions about where we will spend our energy and emotions.

Retail Therapy Beats Chemotherapy

> My advice to you is not to inquire why or
> whither, but just enjoy your ice cream
> while it's on your plate.
> —*Thornton Wilder*

One of my mantras over the course of my treatment was "Whatever it takes, do it." In other words, "This isn't the time to be practical. Whatever it takes to feel better, if it's feasible and legal, do it." And I did. And it helped.

TRIED-AND-TRUE WAYS TO MAKE THINGS A LITTLE BETTER

- Treat yourself to something special after each treatment (assuming you'll feel like it) and decide on it in advance. For example, have "high tea" with a friend, go out for ice cream with another friend, or pick up a magazine that you usually don't buy.

- Keep a cache of fizzling bath salts, beautiful candles, a CD player, and a brand-new fluffy, soft towel in the bathroom and lock yourself in for a relaxing home spa treatment. (T.J. Maxx and Marshalls have indulgent bath products at a discount.)

- Discover the wonderful world of QVC, where you can find things that you didn't even know existed and now can't live without. Truly, it became one of my favorite destinations, and I never got my Christmas shopping done faster or more successfully.

- Plan something special. It's important to make plans, for both the short term and long term. Imaging and visualization are important tools for promoting health, and that includes visualizing and anticipating special events, both large and small—things like a cruise, a few days at a spa, a splurge at your favorite store, a trip to a foreign country, or a trip to The Body Shop.

I decided that I wanted to take a fancy cruise with my husband along the Mediterranean coast to celebrate the return of my hair. I spent countless hours researching the possibilities and finally came up with the perfect trip. I got so much satisfaction and pleasure from planning it that when we ended up canceling (for unrelated reasons) I hardly felt deprived: it almost seemed to me as if I'd taken it!

PLANET CANCER OR "DO I REALLY NEED TO SEE A COUNSELOR?"

When I was diagnosed, I felt as if my body had betrayed me. In fact, my body suddenly seemed like another entity—part of me, yet at the same time separate. "Who are you? How could you do this?" I'd ask it. "We've been together for forty-seven years. I thought I knew you. I thought you liked me!" I felt alone in a way that I could hardly describe. I was in uncharted territory—Planet Cancer, I called it—and as much as others loved and supported me, they couldn't be there with me.

On Earth, I knew how to navigate through my life pretty well. But on Planet Cancer I was constantly tripping over one new fear or another: physical fears, the fear of being a burden, concerns about how my family would be affected by my illness, financial concerns, not to mention some anger and resentment.

Being a big believer in not reinventing the wheel, I decided that if there were ways to handle having cancer that had already been devised, then I'd rather not try to come up with them myself.

In therapy, I learned new ways to deal with many of my fears and upsets that have served me well long after my illness passed. I also learned that, unlike most any other place, you never need to censor yourself in a therapist's office in order to protect other people or to hide reactions that you think are "unacceptable."

And if you're fortunate enough to find a therapist as extraordinary as mine, then you may well find that it's the one doctor's appointment that you actually look forward to.

THE VALUE OF JOURNALING

Apart from counseling, writing in my journal was the most helpful way of uncovering, sorting through, and examining all the "stuff" that was dropping into my life like asteroids on Planet Cancer. Like counseling, my journal was a safe place to express everything I was feeling, and I often found that the very process of writing clarified why I was worried about a particular thing or how I'd handle a situation the next time it arose.

Studies at major institutions around the country, including Ohio State University, Southern Methodist University, and M. D. Anderson Cancer Center, have determined that the practice of writing provides the following overall health benefits: pain reduction, immune function improvement (including increase in T cell counts), resistance to minor illnesses such as colds and the flu, and lower blood pressure and heart rate. The connections between writing and increased physical well-being are so interesting to the medical community that the National Institutes of Health is sponsoring a five-year study to examine the physical and psychological benefits of counseling and journaling in cancer patients.

Getting Started

Buy an inexpensive notebook to write in. Don't buy a fancy blank book. Spiral is an easier format for writing; more important, fancy books can be very intimidating and become obstacles to writing. If typing is easier; keep your journal in your computer. This is not for an audience or for publication. This is for your eyes and your use. You might never want to share it, and that's fine.

- If anybody else uses your computer, consider using a boring alias for the file, such as "Physics" or "Cleaning Supplies." Nobody will be tempted to peek!

- Because starting a journal can be daunting, give yourself permission to write for just five minutes. You can do anything for five minutes. If you want to stop then, no problem. Chances are, though, that once you start writing, the time will fly.

- If you haven't kept a journal before, it may be a little intimidating to start. After you get the hang of it, you won't have to think about what you're going to write about. For now, here are a couple of suggestions just to get you going. First, you've been through an awful lot in a short time. What's happened up until now? How did you learn about your diagnosis? How have you been surprised by how people have responded to the news? What treatment(s) are you having? How are you getting along with your medical team? How do you feel about what's happened to you? Remember, be honest. This journal is for your eyes only.

Keeping a journal serves a number of purposes: it's the chronicle of a time in your life like no other. Hard as it is to believe, the time will come when you don't remember as much of this marathon as you expect to now.

Perhaps most important, this inanimate object that probably cost only a few dollars will gradually become your confidant. You'll be able to tell it things that you may not tell anyone else. By telling those things, you'll probably gain insights and even some answers to some very thorny issues. Silly as it may sound, your journal will become an intimate friend.

HANDLING THE HOLIDAYS

The bottom line for handling the holiday season is: do—or don't do—whatever you need to in order to get through it. That might mean sleeping through it if you don't have little ones or pets. There aren't any good one-size-fits-all answers to the holiday issue, but here are a few tactics that can help a bit:

- Accept an invitation or two if you're up to it. It really is better to be with other people than to be sitting alone in your living room. Don't feel obligated to accept all invitations—or even most. Just don't be a hermit.

- Take a vacation from the busy work associated with holidays. This is the year that you can get away with anything, so do what you want to do and forget the rest. It'll all be there for you to do next year. If you don't want to send out cards, don't.

- If you do want to send out cards, donate to a charity that will send out holiday cards to your list, with a note in each card indicating that you've made a donation in the person's name. Then you'll have taken care of cards and gifts. (This can get expensive, so be choosy.)

- If you're buying gifts, find something on the Internet or QVC that most anyone would like—a little flashlight, a purse pen—and then buy ten or twenty of them. Give them to everyone on your list (within reason).

- By now, you know for sure that it isn't presents or parties or fattening foods that give the holidays their meaning, so don't feel pressured to do anything except be with the people you love (on your terms, of course).

humor—it really is the best medicine

(well, at least it doesn't make you nauseous)

> Show me a patient who is able to laugh and play, who enjoys living and I'll show you someone who is going to live longer. Laughter makes the unbearable bearable, and a patient with a well-developed sense of humor has a better chance of recovery than a stolid individual who seldom laughs.
> —*Dr. Bernie Siegel*
> *Author of* Love, Miracles and Medicine

> To succeed in life you need three things: a wishbone, a backbone, and a funny bone.
> —*Reba McEntire*

What's Funny about Cancer?

That's easy. The answer is NOTHING. There's nothing even mildly amusing about cancer, much less funny. But there are books, scientific studies from prestigious universities, and powerful first-person accounts that attest to the healing power of humor. Not curing power, but healing power.

When you laugh, your chest, abdominal muscles, diaphragm, and lungs contract, giving your body the equivalent of a mini workout. Your heart rate and blood pressure increase as if you were doing aerobic exercise. Adrenaline is pumped into your blood, and endorphins are released.

Medical science has found that endorphins trigger "runner's high," a sort of euphoria, and help strengthen the immune system. It's also established that laughter increases antibodies, activates T immune cells, and decreases stress hormones, and that laughter helps to decrease pain by causing physical relaxation and reducing anxiety.

In the movie *Patch Adams*, based on a true story, Robin Williams plays a young physician whose extraordinary use of fun, humor, and laughter transforms the attitudes of seriously ill patients of all ages. If you haven't seen it, do.

Some hospitals are introducing "humor rooms" in their oncology wings, which include players for comedy DVDs, games, toys, costumes, NERF balls, and bubbles. And they're on the adult floors.

So even though there's nothing funny about having cancer, there are reasons to see the humor in life, even some of the ironic, outrageous situations that arise from being in this pickle. Don't forgo any opportunity to laugh that comes along.

Jokes Only a Cancer Patient Could Love

A doctor tells his patient, "The tests show your cancer is advanced. You have six months to live." "But, Doctor, I can't pay off my medical bills in six months," the patient exclaims. "In that case," says the doctor, "you have a year."

A doctor finally reaches his patient after several days of phone tag to report the results of his medical tests. "Do you want the good news or the bad news?" he asks. "The good news," the patient replies. "You have forty-eight hours to live," says the doctor. "That's the good news?" cries the patient. "What could possibly be the bad news?" "I called last week."

Paul and Jack, two old baseball buddies, both with cancer, are chatting on a park bench. "I hope they have a baseball team in heaven," says the first. "Me, too," his friend replies. "Tell you what, if I die first, I'll give you a message about whether there's baseball in heaven. If you die first, you can do the same for me," he suggests. A year later, Paul is dead and Jack is on the park bench. He hears "Jack, it's me, Paul. I have great news! There really is a baseball team in heaven." "Thank God," Jack says, "now I can die in peace." "I'm glad you feel that way," Paul says, "because you're pitching tomorrow."

Q: What do you call a young woman who keeps getting lymphoma over and over again?

A: A lymphomaniac.

A very religious woman is diagnosed with cancer. Certain that God will heal her, she turns down treatment from a cancer surgeon, a radiologist, and an oncologist. She soon dies and the first thing she says to God is "I believed in you. I thought you were going to heal me. What happened?" "Got me!" says God. "I sent you a surgeon, a radiologist, and an oncologist!"

Movies Guaranteed to Make You Laugh

Tootsie
Ghostbusters
Blazing Saddles (or any Mel Brooks movie)
Little Miss Sunshine
Trading Places

EIGHT WAYS YOU KNOW YOUR DOCTOR IS AN ONCOLOGIST

1 He asks you if you want to have a port, and he's not offering you a drink.

2 Even though he is wearing a white lab coat and not a military uniform, he keeps using words like "battle," "fight," "war," and "weapons."

3 He tries to explain to you why a low grade is better than a high grade on your report.

4 He talks a lot about trials, and, as far as you know, he's not a lawyer or a judge.

5 When he shakes hands with you at your initial appointment, you have a feeling that he's checking you out.

6 He tells you that you will get a series of treatments and you keep wondering where the facial and massage part comes in.

7 He tells you that you are on a protocol and it doesn't seem to fit with the dictionary definition (a form of ceremony and etiquette observed by diplomats and heads of state).

8 He has you sign a consent form for treatment that's more intimidating than the diagnosis.

POSITIVE THINGS ABOUT NOT HAVING HAIR (NOT A HUGE LIST)

1 The shower and sink drains require a lot less Drano.

2 You now prefer hair-raising movies.

3 You can remove your hair when you weigh yourself.

4 People can see a strong resemblance between you and your new grandchild.

5 You don't have to wash your hair.

6 If you go to the bowling alley and there's a long wait for a lane, just put your turban on, place your bowling ball in front of you and charge for fortune readings.

7 You don't have to shave your legs (or your chin).

8 You don't have to worry about your bikini line.

9 If you walk through the airport in your bathrobe without your wig, people will give you money. The best airport, according to my sources, is in San Francisco.

well-meaning family, friends, and strangers

Your Spouse

Not to play one-upmanship, but did I mention that four years after I was diagnosed with cancer, my husband learned that he had prostate cancer? Until then, I'd considered myself the cancer expert in residence. But my experience as his caregiver showed me a side of cancer I hadn't expected. For example, what could be worse than being nauseous, bald, bandaged, green, in pain, and exhausted? I'm not sure. But watching someone you love be nauseous, bald, bandaged, green, in pain, and exhausted—and not being able to do anything about it—is right up there.

Here are a few things that you and your partner can do for each other that will help bring you through this closer than you were before:

- Remember that he's feeling as frightened, besieged, and overwhelmed as you are. Even though you need for him to be strong, cut him some slack. You've both been hit by a two-ton truck.

- Stay in touch with each other. Make sure that you *keep talking* to each other about how you're both faring. Many couples do this as the last thing each night before they go to sleep.

- Make sure that your partner attends to his own needs as well as yours and your family's. Don't let him burn out.

- Say "thank you" and "I love you" every day, not just to your spouse, but to all those who are in this with you.

- Use the support services offered by your hospital/cancer center and by organizations like the American Cancer Society and CancerCare. They have professional counselors for caregivers who are always available as well as caregiver support groups.

Your Parents

It doesn't matter that you're an adult; maybe you're a parent yourself, or even a grandparent. But no matter how old you are, you'll always be Mommy's and Daddy's little girl—which is one of the many reasons why it's so *especially* difficult to bring parents into the loop. There are few things more painful than to have to watch one's child suffer a devastating illness.

Some people's relationship with one or both parents remains complicated long past childhood. If your mother was overprotective when you were a child, you shudder to think how she'll hover now. No matter what the nature of your relationship with your parents is, it will intensify as you fight this illness. To keep everybody in check:

- Remember that you're a grown-up now. You can accept as much—or as little—help and/or advice from your parents as you want. And you can say, "No thank you," too.

- Stay honest. Your parents want to know the real scoop. Don't underplay what's going on in order to spare them. Remember, they're grown-ups too.

Your Children

If you have children, then you have yet another layer of concern to cope with. As most cancer help organizations will tell you, the best thing you can do is tell your children what's happening to the degree that they're able to take it in and handle it. As you well know, children have great instincts, and yours are going to know early on that something's up. Just like adults, the less they understand, the more their vivid imaginations will take over and cause them to get more upset than if they were brought into the loop. It will be far better for them and for you if you tell them—sooner rather than later—and allow them to do things that will make them feel that they're helping you get better.

The good news is that you don't have to go it alone. Cancer*Care*, which offers many wonderful services, has a program called Cancer*Care* for Kids. It's a staff of professional oncology social workers who offer you support and advice and will counsel your children to help them understand what's happening, either via telephone, online, or in person (www.cancercare.org; 800-HOPE).

Cancer*Care*'s Ten Tips for Communicating with Your Children

1. Give your children accurate, age-appropriate information about cancer. Don't be afraid to use the word "cancer" and tell them where it is in the body. Practice your explanation beforehand so you feel more comfortable. If you don't provide this information for them, they will often invent their own explanations, which can be even more frightening than the facts.

2. Explain the treatment plan and what this will mean to them (for example, Bobby's mom will be bringing you to soccer practice for a while). Prepare your children for any physical changes you might encounter throughout treatment (hair loss, weight gain or loss, fatigue, and so on).

3. Answer your children's questions as accurately as possible and appropriately for their ages and prior experience with serious illness in the family. If you do not know the answer to a question, don't panic. Say, "I don't know. I will try to find out the answer."

4. Comfort your children by explaining that no matter how they have been behaving or what their thoughts have been, they did not do anything to cause the cancer. Explain that they cannot "catch" cancer as they can catch a cold.

5. Let your children know about other members of the support system, including your partner, relatives, friends, clergy, teachers, coaches, and your health care team. Let them know they can ask these adults questions and can always talk to them about their feelings.

6. Allow your children to participate in and make a contribution to your care by giving them age-appropriate tasks, such as bringing you a glass of water or reading to you.

7. Encourage your children to express their feelings, even ones that are uncomfortable. But also let them know it's okay to say "I don't want to talk right now."

8. Assure your children that their needs are still important and that they will be cared for, even if you can't always provide the care directly.

9. Spend your energy communicating with your children. Understand what they are asking, even if you can't always provide the care directly.

10. As always, show them lots of love and affection. Let them know that although things are different, your love for them has not changed.

Friends, Strangers, and Answers to "How Can I Help?"

First, tell people how they can help. It sounds simple, but for many of us it's very difficult to let others do things for us. If there's ever a time when you need to get over that, it's now.

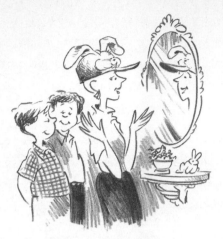

"OH, TIMMY...BROOKS! IT'S SO ME!"

It's very important to realize that other people really want to help you through this. And when they ask what you need, they mean it. You'll make it easier for them and for you if you're clear and specific about what would help you. If you need to make cupcakes for your child's class, ask somebody to do that for you. If you need someone to help you change your nightgown, ask a friend you're comfortable with. Trust me, if people aren't serious about being there for you, they won't ask again.

The next few pages are intended for you to copy and give to everyone who will be helping you, including your spouse. Like all the information in this book, it is the result of many people's experience and is guaranteed to make your life a lot easier. Besides, by giving it to others, it will spare you from telling people things that are better conveyed by someone else.

TRIED-AND-TRUE WAYS TO BEST HELP YOUR FRIEND

It is one of the most beautiful compensations of this life that no man can sincerely try to help another without also helping himself.

—*Ralph Waldo Emerson*

If you're reading this, then you're an important person in your friend's life. She has just been drafted into a battle for which she hasn't been trained. But she knows that there are some people who will help her through this war, and you're one of them.

I fought the same war a few years ago, and I couldn't have done it without people like you who were there for me. During that time I realized that just as I had no instruction manual for fighting my battle, my friends didn't have a manual to go by either.

Below are some guidelines for you as you help your friend. They're intended to help you keep from burning out, too. After all, that's the best way to help your friend.

Good Things to Say

- I'm so sorry this is happening to you.

- I'm thinking of and praying for you every day.

- You're going to get through this, and I'll be with you along the way.

- When you're better (as opposed to "if you get better") . . .

Tried-and-True Ways to Help

- Remember that you're *not* a statistic.

- I can only imagine how hard this must be for you to go through (not "I know how hard this is for you").

- Please know that I'm here for you. Anytime you want to talk about anything, please let me know.

- I don't know what to say, but I want you to know that I care.

What Not to Say

- You're the last person I would have expected to get cancer.

- What's your prognosis?

- If you had to have cancer, this is the best one to get.

Rule of Thumb

Put yourself in your friend's place and imagine that someone was saying this to you. If it would make you feel better, then say it. If you wouldn't want to hear it, don't say it.

Good Things to Do for Your Friend

- Tell her—*don't ask* her—what you're going to do. For example, tell her that you're going to bring over dinner or a frozen casserole, or schedule rides for her to and from treatments. You can always add, "Or is there something else that would be more helpful to you now?" This is much more helpful than asking the well-intentioned-but-less-helpful open-ended "What can I do?"

- Bring food in disposable containers.

- CALL FIRST. Any time you want to drop something off or visit, find out what would be a good time for you to come by.

- Take your cues from her. She may want to talk about it a lot, or she may want to be more reticent. The main thing you can do for her is to let her know that you care.

- When you come by to pick up the kids, etc., DO NOT STAY—even for a cup of coffee—unless she begs you to.

- If you do visit at her invitation, don't stay long.

- *Err on the side of too short rather than too long a visit.* The gift of several brief visits is far better than that of one long one.

- Don't be afraid to hug or touch your friend as you did before she was diagnosed. She won't break, and she's probably feeling pretty isolated by now and could use a good hug.

- When in doubt, e-mail instead of calling, especially if your friend doesn't have an answering machine.

Tried-and-True Ways to Help

- Be sensitive about which books you give as gifts. Don't give or even recommend cancer memoirs unless your friend asks for one. Later on, she'll be more inspired by others' stories of overcoming their battles, but right now she's busy fighting her own battle.

- Don't tell your friend about other people you know who had cancer, even if they're better now.

- Coordinate car pool rides for her children.

- Drive her to treatments and offer to stay with her during treatment. You can probably go in and keep her company, which will not only comfort her, but it'll make the time fly.

- Offer to care for her children when she has medical appointments.

- Don't come to visit in groups, even as small as two people.

- Don't send flowers now. Do it later to celebrate milestones like the end of treatment or the first hair to appear on her head.

- Don't bring lotions if your friend is having radiation; her skin will be sensitive to many ingredients in most lotions and creams.

Tried-and-True Ways to Help

- Consider waiting for a few weeks after her diagnosis or surgery before bringing her a get-well token or present. By then the attention will have died down a little, and your gesture will mean that much more to her.

- Keep your friend as involved and in the loop as possible. Include her in social events and projects. She probably won't participate much, but she'll feel as if she's still a full-fledged part of the group, and that's what's most important.

- Don't offer unsolicited advice or opinions.

- Don't spend time with her or her family if you have a cold or even the sniffles. Her immune system is pretty much gone.

- Don't be patronizing. It's easy to slip into the singsong "So-how's-the-patient?" mode. But that will make your friend feel even more helpless than she already does.

Gifts Guaranteed to Please

- *Never underestimate the value of a card!* Send cards often throughout your friend's treatment. Buy a few at a time and address and stamp the envelopes so you can pop them in the mail frequently. No need for long notes—a simple "thinking of you" works wonders. By the way, e-cards are nice, but nothing takes the place of ripping into an envelope that's just arrived.

- Organize a card shower, which is just a fancy term for getting a lot of people to send cards. One e-mail to as many of her friends and colleagues as you can locate is all it takes. Just be sure to include her address. Since it's more fun to get cards on an ongoing basis than in one fell swoop, you all don't need to send them at once. When it comes to receiving cards, there's no such thing as too late.

- Buy her a subscription to a magazine she wouldn't normally get for herself, or give her a few of your recent issues.

- Give her a gift certificate to a local restaurant or bookstore, or for babysitting services for an evening.

- Combine the two above certificates to create a "date night" with another friend; it will be an extremely welcome treat.

- Offer to set up a Web site for her where friends can write notes and get updates.

- If you're paperwork-oriented, help with health care claims.

Tried-and-True Ways to Help

- Prepare a bag of goodies for your friend to take to appointments and treatment. Include such items as a magazine, water bottle, hard candy, pen and pad, and even a small pillow or micro fleece throw.

Other great gifts you can give include little stones or medallions engraved with words such as "healing" and "serenity" or other uplifting words (I was given one and carried it in my pocket—whenever I was out of my robe!), a pretty silk scarf square if your friend has lost her hair, music and meditation CDs, a prepaid long-distance telephone calling card, earplugs and an eye mask for sleeping, a small handheld fan with foam blades (for the woman in menopause), a set of pretty blank note cards and stamps, or two hours devoted to doing anything she'd like done for her.

But the best gift of all is simply being there and listening. There's no need to talk. Remember: you don't need to solve the problem. If you could, there'd be a Nobel Prize in your future.

Most important of all: don't take on too much (since you're in this for the long haul, you need to make sure you don't burn out. Be sure to pace yourself) . . . so you won't disappear. It's far better to stay involved in a way that doesn't drain you than to exhaust yourself and become unable to continue to be there for your friend.

staying home and going out

Regardless of what your job situation is, it's important to remember that *you have a new full-time job: you're a CEO*. Not only that, you aren't putting in an eight- or ten- or twelve-hour day; you're spending 24/7 on this job. And on top of everything else, you're doing all this with diminished energy and strength, not to mention those annoying things like nausea, loss of appetite, and anxiety. You're now working two jobs when it's harder than it was to do just one.

Not many of us have the luxury of taking an unpaid leave of absence, although many employers are legally bound to provide one for a designated period of time. If you have disability insurance, you may be eligible for short- or long-term disability benefits. Even if you think you know what the answer is, check with your employer. It would be a shame if you were to miss out on benefits you assumed you didn't have.

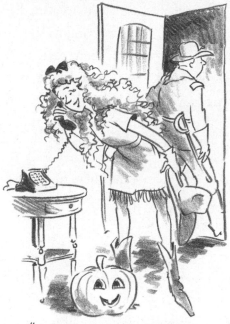

"TO A COSTUME PARTY... I'M GOING AS A PERSON WITH HAIR!"

Staying Home

It sounds obvious, but do as little housework as possible. Don't straighten up when people visit; they aren't thinking about what your house looks like.

ATTRACTIVE HOME WEAR HINTS

- Whether you're greeting company or just getting

the mail, glance in the mirror before you open the door. Not to make sure you're wearing lipstick—or even your robe. I'm just trying to spare you from opening the door and then remembering, not necessarily right away, that you're not wearing anything on your bald head. (If, on the other hand, you don't want a return visit from that particular person, it's probably a good idea.)

- Keep a scarf or cap somewhere near the front door so you can put it on at the last minute when the doorbell rings.

- Invest in a good robe and slippers. You'll be getting much more use out of them than almost anything else (except your pj's), and not because you'll be feeling so sick—you'll just want to be as comfortable as possible.

- If you're entertaining guests at home and want to dress up, comparatively speaking, several sets of yoga clothes provide both comfort and style.

- If you've been put into menopause thanks to your treatment, keep a couple of extra nightgowns by your bed, since you may well want to change in the middle of the night due to "the sweats."

ENTERTAINING VISITORS (WHO'S THE SICK ONE HERE?)

People have the best of intentions, but they don't always know what isn't appropriate. That said, it is not your job to educate them or indulge them if you don't feel like accepting their visit right then. Your job is to rest, conserve your energy, and take care of your needs. You can be gracious and firm; they'll understand. If you're not up to having visitors, some things you can do include the following:

- Just say no.

- Use the "good cop/bad cop" routine. If possible, have your spouse or partner answer the phone or the door and say, "She'd love to see you, but she's resting."

- Invest in Caller ID. Use it to screen calls.

- Feel free to ignore your e-mail's "instant messaging," or check to see if you can change your availability icon on-screen. Some e-mail programs let you set your availability as "busy."

- Don't answer the door if somebody rings your doorbell unannounced.

When you're up for company, here are some things you can do to save energy and enjoy your visit more:

- Pretend you're the guest. Try not to start fixing plates of cookies and cups of coffee for your company. They aren't here because they're hungry, and they certainly don't want to put you to work. If you feel you must offer refreshments, say something like "The tea bags are in the canister if you'd like to make yourself a cup."

- Don't get dressed. Seriously. Stay in your pj's and robe if you want to make sure that your guests remember just why they're there. It's a constant, silent reminder that your body is at war and it's tired.

- Have an exit strategy. There's nothing worse than being ready for your guests to leave before they are. If you have your "out" planned in advance, you'll enjoy the visit much more knowing that you won't be needing to figure out a tactful way to say it's time to leave.

My father used to say, "It's time for me to go to bed so that you all can go home." I opted for a less-blunt approach. The best exit strategy I found was to tell my guests in advance that I was delighted they were coming, but I had an appointment and would have to end the visit at X o'clock. (People will usually assume that your "appointment" is with a doctor, but in my case, it was often just with my down comforter and DVD player. But it was an appointment, right?) This worked like a charm every time. Humbling as it was, I also realized that my guests were relieved to have an exit strategy, too!

Making the Most of Going Out

During my treatment, I'd have been happy to stay home most all the time. Not because I felt so ill (I felt surprisingly well for most of it), but because my energy was definitely limited and my bald head always required some attention. But how many of us have the option to stay in? Certainly I didn't.

I had to go to work, doctors' appointments, grocery shopping . . . in other words, life went on. Which is actually a good thing. After all, that's exactly what I was fighting for.

TIPS FOR GOING OUT

- Rule of thumb: dress for yourself, not for others. If it makes you feel better to wear makeup and heels, do it. But if you don't . . .

- This is your chance to "go casual." If you're still working, dress nicely, but you don't have to be a fashion plate. If you're going to someone's house for dinner, wear something comfortable. If there was ever a time when nobody's concerned about whether your shoes match your outfit, it's now.

- Piggyback errands you must do. Keep a running list of errands you need to do so that when you go out, you can be most efficient.

- Let others do errands for you; save your energy for the things you want or have to do.

- Ask a friend to drive you to do your errands. This is a great way to take advantage of people's offers to help. And think of all the energy you'll save just by not having to find parking spaces.

top (approximately) ten . . .

Things to Do While Waiting . . .

1 *to see the doctor*
Write thank-you notes.

2 *to see the doctor again*
Catch up in your journal.

3 *to start your next round of chemo*
Take up a crossword puzzle or sudoku.

4 *for your next round of radiation*
Start working on your holiday gift list; it's never too early.

5 *for a CT scan*
Breathe a brief prayer for those who are there for you, doing their best to help make this all a little easier for you.

6 *for a bout of nausea to pass*

Sorry, I can't help you out there. Do whatever it takes.

7 *for your prescription*

Pretend you're a guest on *Oprah*. Let her interview you about what you're going through. Give her your own advice for getting through cancer treatment with your sanity intact. Who knows? Maybe she'll invite you back.

8 *to finish a round of chemo*

Decide what you're going to treat yourself to after your next round of chemo (you know what you're treating yourself to after this one, right?).

9 *for your hair to grow back*

Think about how you can thank the people who've been there for you after life gets back to normal (and remember that it will). You may want to have a tea after your treatment is over and give your guests a small token of your gratitude.

10 *for your ride*

Nothing. Do nothing. Close your eyes, breathe, be still.

Music to Have Chemo By

1 "I Run for Life," Melissa Etheridge

2 Brandenburg Concertos 1–6, J. S. Bach

3 Piano Concerto No. 21 in C Major ("Elvira Madigan"), W. A. Mozart

4 *Frank Sinatra: The Best of the Capitol Years*

5 *Duets: An American Classic*, Tony Bennett

6 *Kind of Blue*, Miles Davis

7 *Feels Like Home*, Norah Jones

8 *We Shall Overcome: The Seeger Sessions*, Bruce Springsteen

9 *Into White*, Carly Simon

10 *Awake*, Josh Groban

11 *Unplugged*, Eric Clapton

Movies to Entertain and Distract

There's a reason why the phrase "mind over matter" has been around for so long: it's true. I found that watching movies (as long as they weren't tear-jerkers) was one of the best ways to take a mental break from my body. Here are some great ones.

GENERAL

1 *The Italian Job* (1969 version, starring Michael Caine and Noel Coward)

2 *When Harry Met Sally*

3 *To Kill a Mockingbird*

4 *Rear Window*

5 *Bridget Jones's Diary*

6 *Patch Adams*

7 *Butch Cassidy and the Sundance Kid*

8 *Because of Winn-Dixie*

9 *Finding Nemo*

10 *The Godfather* (I and II)

COMEDIES

1 Some Like It Hot

2 The Blues Brothers

3 The Pink Panther (1963, starring Peter Sellers)

4 The Producers (1968, starring Zero Mostel and Gene Wilder)

5 Young Frankenstein

6 City Slickers

7 A Night at the Opera

8 Bringing Up Baby

9 The Jerk

10 The African Queen

MUSICALS

1 The Wizard of Oz

2 Little Shop of Horrors

3 Oliver!

4 The Phantom of the Opera

5 Guys and Dolls

6 *Show Boat*

7 *Grease*

8 *My Fair Lady*

9 *The King and I*

10 *Funny Girl*

Novels to Make Time Fly

1 *The Devil Wears Prada*, Lauren Weisberger

2 *Harry Potter and the Sorcerer's Stone*, J. K. Rowling

3 *Memoirs of a Geisha*, Arthur Golden

4 *Bridget Jones's Diary*, Helen Fielding

5 *The Stone Diaries*, Carol Shields

6 *Anna Karenina*, Leo Tolstoy (It's very long, but an incredible love story.)

7 *The Gold Coast*, Nelson DeMille

8 *To Kill a Mockingbird*, Harper Lee

9 *The Good Earth*, Pearl S. Buck

10 *The Kite Runner*, Khaled Hosseini

Helpful Cancer Books

1 *It's Not About the Bike: My Journey Back to Life,* Lance Armstrong

2 *Breast Cancer Husband: How to Help Your Wife (and Yourself) Through Diagnosis, Treatment, and Beyond,* Marc Silver (This book is extremely helpful for couples, regardless of the type of cancer diagnosis.)

3 *When It's Cancer: The 10 Essential Steps to Follow After Your Diagnosis,* Toni Bernay and Saar Porrath

4 *Getting Well Again,* O. Carl Simonton and Stephanie Matthews-Simonton

5 *Every Second Counts,* Lance Armstrong

6 *Cancer Vixen: A True Story,* Marisa Acocella Marchetto

7 *Why I Wore Lipstick to My Mastectomy,* Geralyn Lucas

8 *Love, Medicine and Miracles,* Bernie S. Siegel

9 *Happiness in a Storm: Facing Illness and Embracing Life as a Healthy Survivor,* Wendy Schlessel Harpham

10 *Saving Graces,* Elizabeth Edwards

Cancer Web Sites

These Web sites are not in order of preference; they are all excellent and offer different types of services and information.

1 www.cancercare.org (Cancer*Care*)

2 www.cancer.org (American Cancer Society)

3 www.mdanderson.org (M. D. Anderson Cancer Center)

4 www.patientadvocate.org (Patient Advocate Foundation)

5 www.livestrong.org (The Lance Armstrong Foundation)

6 www.gildasclub.com (Gilda's Club Worldwide)

7 www.mskcc.org (Memorial Sloan-Kettering Cancer Center)

8 www.komen.org (Susan G. Komen Breast Cancer Foundation)

9 www.acor.org (Association of Cancer Online Resources)

10 www.dfci.harvard.edu (Dana Farber Cancer Institute)

11 www.mayoclinic.org (Mayo Clinic)

12 www.cancer.gov (National Cancer Institute)

Myths about Cancer

1 If cancer information is on the printed page, then it's true.

2 If cancer information is on the Internet, then it's true.

3 If the lump hurts, it isn't cancer.

4 The risk of dying from cancer in the U.S. is increasing.

5 Household bug spray can cause cancer.

6 You can prevent skin cancer by applying sunscreen once every day.

7 Some cancer surgeries can cause more harm than good.

8 Antiperspirants or deodorants can cause breast cancer.

9 Everyone with the same kind of cancer gets the same kind of treatment.

10 Drinking coffee increases your chances of getting breast cancer.

Bible Passages to Comfort and Encourage

1 Jeremiah 29:11 "'For I know the plans I have for you,' declares the LORD, 'plans to prosper you and not to harm you, plans to give you a hope and a future.'"

2 Psalm 121 "I lift up my eyes to the hills—where does my help come from? My help comes from the LORD, the Maker of heaven and earth. He will not let your foot slip—he who watches over you will not slumber; indeed, he who watches over Israel will neither slumber nor sleep. The LORD watches over you—the LORD is your shade at your right hand; the sun will not harm you by day, nor the moon by night. The LORD will keep you from all harm—he will watch over your life; the LORD will watch over your coming and going both now and forevermore."

3 Isaiah 40:31 "But those who hope in the LORD will renew their strength. They will soar on wings like eagles; they will run and not grow weary, and they will walk, and not be faint."

4 Psalm 23 "The LORD is my shepherd; I shall not be in want. He makes me lie down in green pastures, he leads me beside quiet waters, he restores my soul. He guides me in the paths of righteousness for his name's sake. Even though I walk through the valley of the shadow of death, I will fear no evil, for you are with me; your rod and your staff, they comfort me. You prepare a table before me in the presence of my enemies. You anoint my head with oil; my cup overflows. Surely goodness and love will follow me all the days of my life, and I will dwell in the house of the LORD forever."

5 John 16:33 "I have told you these things, so that in me you may have peace. In this world you will have trouble. But take heart! I have overcome the world."

6 Matthew 10:29–31 "Are not two sparrows sold for a penny? Yet not one of them will fall to the ground apart from the will of your Father. And even the very hairs of your head are all numbered. So don't be afraid; you are worth more than many sparrows."

7 Psalm 91:1–7 "He who dwells in the shelter of the Most High will rest in the shadow of the Almighty. I will say of the LORD, 'He is my refuge and my fortress, my God, in whom I trust.' Surely he will save you from the fowler's snare and from the deadly pestilence. He will cover you with his feathers, and under his wings you will find refuge; his faithfulness will be your shield and rampart. You will not fear the terror of night, nor the arrow that flies by day, nor the pestilence that stalks in the darkness, nor the plague that destroys at midday. A thousand may fall at your side, ten thousand at your right hand, but it will not come near you."

8 I Peter 5:7 "Cast all your anxiety on him because he cares for you."

9 Matthew 11:28–30 "Come to me, all you who are weary and burdened, and I will give you rest. Take my yoke upon you and learn from me, for I am gentle and humble in heart, and you will find rest for your souls. For my yoke is easy and my burden is light."

10 Daniel 6:23 "And when Daniel was lifted from the [lions'] den, no wound was found on him, because he had trusted in his God."

Things to Remember When You're Really Down

1 This, too, shall pass.

2 You are NOT a statistic.

3 The day is coming when cancer won't dominate your thinking, time, energy, and your life (really and truly).

4 You're not in this alone. You're surrounded by people who would do anything for you except probably take your place. (But you can't blame them for that.)

5 and **6** and **7**. There are still things to be grateful for. Think of three.

8 A year from today, this will be behind you.

9 You're probably facing the hardest thing you'll ever have to deal with. So it can get only better from here.

Things Others Can Do to Help That Take Less Than Thirty Minutes

1 Run the vacuum.

2 Take your kids out for a soda (for a change of pace for everybody).

3 Put a load of laundry into your washer.

4 Put a load of laundry into your dryer.

5 Straighten out the refrigerator contents (and toss some if necessary).

6 Make some sandwiches, snacks, or lunches ahead for your kids.

7 Separate junk mail from your personal mail, magazines, and catalogs.

8 Help you make a list of people who have been sending things and helping you, so you can acknowledge them after you're better.

9 Bring over a take-out lunch and share it with you.

10 Unload the dishwasher.

Good Things That Will Happen as a Result of Chemo

1 Thick, lush hair on your head will replace your old hair.

2 Lavish curls will replace old straight hair, followed by new straight hair as your curly hair grows out.

3 You will never take your hair on your head and eyebrows, nose hair, and pubic hair for granted again.

4 When something goes wrong and you say "It could be worse," you mean it.

5 No more hair on your legs (in some cases).

6 No more hair under your arms (in some cases).

7 Your skin will look like someone's who is twenty years younger than you.

8 You can say, "Sorry, I'm just not up to it," even if you are, for at least the next several months.

9 You'll never wish you didn't have an appetite.

10 You won't take everyday things for granted.

complementary, integrative, and alternative treatments

Until about twenty years ago, the scientific medical community didn't accept or recognize nontraditional, natural remedies and approaches to healing as having value. But now there's a growing movement to integrate traditional and nontraditional approaches to healing called "complementary" or "integrative" therapy, and many cancer centers are offering integrative therapies along with conventional medical treatment. Alternative medicine is defined by the American Cancer Society as all those unproven methods that are offered as cures and are used instead of conventional therapies.

It's estimated that almost 80 percent of cancer patients use at least one nontraditional therapy during their course of treatment.

Some of the most common complementary therapies include acupuncture, used for pain and nausea; healing touch; massage; yoga; meditation; journaling; guided imagery; reflexology; Pilates; tai chi; and dance, music, and art therapies. Integrative medicine uses therapies that include biofeedback, chiropractors, clergy, exercise trainers, herbal protocols, massage, pharmacologists, meditation and relaxation techniques, physical therapists, physicians who specialize in complementary and integrative medicine, physical therapy, and psychologists or psychiatrists.

Complementary and alternative medicine are different from each other, even though they're often discussed in tandem. Complementary medicine (also called integrative medicine) is used *together with* conventional/standard medicine. Alternative medicine is used *in place of* conventional/standard medicine.

The types of complementary/alternative medicine (CAM) include:

- Mind-body interventions, which include meditation, prayer, imaging, journaling, and therapies such as art, music, and dance therapy

- Biologically based therapies, which use substances found in nature such as herbs and foods for special diets

- Manipulative and body-based methods, which include massage and chiropractic treatments

- Energy therapy, which focuses on fields around the human body and includes therapeutic touch, Reiki, Qigong.

If you're considering using any CAM therapies, it's important to discuss it with your medical team before you begin. You should ask them:

- What are the benefits of this therapy? The risks?

- Do the benefits outweigh the risks?

- What are the side effects?

- Will any of these practices interfere with my current treatment?

- Do you know of any clinical trials employing these treatments?

You should also find out if your insurance covers some or all of these treatments.

If you decide to pursue CAM, it's important to ask a practitioner these questions before starting treatment:

- What are the specific benefits of the treatment you're recommending?

- What is your educational/training background?

- May I speak with some of your patients who have similar diagnoses?

- Are there potential side effects?

- How will you know whether the treatment is working?

- Will you communicate with my oncologist?

Resources for Further Information

- NCCAM Clearinghouse, the federal government's lead agency for scientific research on CAM, provides information based on scientific studies of complementary and alternative medicine (www. nccam.nih.gov; e-mail: info@nccam.nih.gov).

- National Cancer Institute has a publication, *Thinking About Complementary & Alternative Medicine* (www. cancer.gov/publications).

- M. D. Anderson Cancer Center provides a concise but thorough overview of the complementary therapy programs that are available to people with cancer (www.mdanderson.org/topics/complementary).

9

survivor!

Faith is not a cushion for me to fall back upon; it is my working energy.

—Helen Keller

Saying Good-bye to Treatment

A funny thing happened on the way to finishing up my treatment. I began to get anxious. Actually, I began to dread my upcoming final treatment. As bad as the chemo and all that had gone with it had been, I'd had megadoses of ammunition and rays destroying the cancer cells in my body. Even when I slept, they were busy hunting down and decimating the sinister cells that had invaded my body and my life.

Now I was about to be pushed off into uncharted waters by myself. A friend described it as feeling like a little rowboat being launched onto a lake without oars or a pilot—or an anchor. The other side of the lake was in sight, but suddenly it was up to me to get there by myself. I didn't want to row the boat alone.

When my doctor said, "I'll see you in three months," I wanted to beg him to let me come back before then. "How about if I come back in a few weeks and you can freshen up my chemo?" I wanted to ask him, as if we were talking about a glass of wine.

Nobody was more surprised about these emotions than I was. I'd spent months that felt like years dealing with endless insults to my body and soul. But now that it was time to start to detox, I found myself afraid to say good-bye to chemo.

It was a big relief to learn that my feelings and fears were common. In fact, the American Cancer Society has found that many survivors are surprised by concerns and fears that they hadn't anticipated.

Not only is there a fear of being sent offshore without a rope, but residual side effects of treatment are probably still making you tired, even though you feel as though you need to go back to your normal responsibilities and routines. And there's also a nagging fear that the cancer could come back.

But the brain is a beautiful thing, and these fears are going to recede until someday you'll wake up and you won't think about them for a few minutes. Then half an hour, a few hours, a day . . . Pretty soon you realize you haven't thought about a recurrence for a week!

Everything I Need to Know I Learned in Treatment

Every day is a precious gift
Don't waste today worrying about tomorrow
Unconditional love is a joy to give and a blessing to
    receive
There are no coincidences . . .
God shines through the people we love and guides us
Slow down
Take deep breaths
Believe in miracles
Don't quit
Never give up hope
Doctors and nurses and their families are extraordinary
    people who need our prayers
Prayer is powerful
Everyone should spend at least one day in an oncologist's
    office
Be generous with your praise
Say "thank you" often
Don't allow little things to upset you
We need very few material possessions to live and be
    happy
Smile
Appreciate the humor in life
Hug those around you
Thank God for family and friends who carry you
    through the difficult times

Eat healthy foods
Walk
Take time to listen to children
Have patience
Listen to music; it's healing
Take one day at a time
Stay in the present
Trust in God

—Author Unknown, posted in a waiting room at the
Dana Farber Cancer Institute

Wonder of wonders, one day it occurs to you that you haven't thought about your cancer—or about cancer at all—for quite a while.

This is hard to imagine, I know. When I was in the throes of cancer, I couldn't believe that I'd ever get back to "normal" or that I wouldn't constantly be aware of the fact that cancer had invaded my space.

But don't rely on my word. Ask people you know who have been on this journey. They'll support my claim.

I'm not saying that your life will be the same as before. It won't.

You'll have a special identification with those who are still members of the club—even strangers. If they mention that they have cancer, you won't cringe and remember that you have to be somewhere else. You'll ask what kind of cancer they have, and you'll let them know that you understand, that someday they won't wake up thinking about cancer, and that one day they'll have burned their membership card, too.

glossary

Here is a group of basic cancer terms that you'll probably encounter. They're just a fraction of the four thousand terms defined in the comprehensive *Dictionary of Cancer Terms*, which can be found at the National Cancer Institute Web site: www.cancer.gov/dictionary.

Acute—Describes symptoms or signs that begin and worsen quickly but don't last for a long period of time; not chronic.

Adjuvant therapy—Treatment given after the primary treatment to increase the chances of a cure.

Alternative medicine—Practices used instead of standard medical treatments. Includes megadose vitamins, herbal preparations, acupuncture, massage therapy, magnet therapy, meditation, healing touch, and other spiritual therapies.

Analgesic—Drug that relieves pain.

Anemia—Deficiency of red blood cells.

Asymptomatic—Having no signs or symptoms of disease.

B cell—White blood cell that comes from the bone marrow. As part of the immune system, B cells make antibodies and help fight infections.

Benign—Noncancerous.

Best practice—In medicine, treatment that experts agree is appropriate, accepted, and widely used. Also called standard therapy or standard of care.

Blood cell counts—Test to check the number of red and white blood cells and platelets. Low red blood cell counts cause tiredness. Low white blood cell counts increase the risk of infection. Low platelet counts increase the risk of bruising and bleeding.

Chronic—Describes a disease or condition that persists or progresses over a long period of time.

Clinical trial—Research studies that test new treatment and prevention methods to find out if they are safe, effective, and better than the current standard of care (the best known treatment). Unlike other scientific studies, these employ human beings as subjects instead of animals or laboratory testing.

Combination chemotherapy—Treatment with drugs that kill cancer cells.

Complementary medicine—Form of alternative treatment that is used in addition to standard/conventional treatments. Generally not considered standard medical approaches. May include dietary supplements, megadose vitamins, herbal preparations, special teas, acupuncture, massage therapy, magnet therapy, spiritual healing, and meditation.

Edema—Swelling caused by excess fluid in body tissues.

Grade—The grade of a tumor indicates its probable growth rate and tendency to spread. It depends on how abnormal the cancer cells look under a microscope and how quickly the tumor is likely to grow and spread. Grading systems are different for each type of cancer.

Hand-foot syndrome—Condition marked by pain, swelling, numbness, tingling, or redness of the hands or feet. A side effect of certain anticancer drugs.

Hope—To expect with confidence. To remember that every cancer at every stage has been survived by someone. An essential for every cancer patient.

Hormonal therapy—Treatment that prevents cancer cells from growing by taking advantage of the hormonal needs of these cells.

In situ cancer—Early cancer that has not spread to neighboring tissue.

Invasive cancer—Cancer that has spread beyond the layer of tissue in which it started and is growing in other tissues or parts of the body.

Killer cell—White blood cell that attacks tumor

cells and body cells that have been invaded by foreign substances.

Lesion—Area of abnormal tissue. A lesion may be benign or malignant.

Localized—Restricted to the site of origin, without evidence of spread.

Localized cancer—Cancer that is confined entirely to the area where it started and has not spread to other parts of the body.

Local therapy—Treatment that affects cells in the tumor and the area close to it.

Lymph, lymph fluid—Clear fluid that travels through the lymphatic system and carries cells that help fight infections and other diseases.

Lymph glands, lymph nodes—Pea-size organs that are located throughout the body. They filter out foreign substances and produce antibodies. Lymph glands filter lymph and store lymphocytes (white blood cells).

Lymphedema—Swelling in the arms or legs caused by excess fluid collected in tissues. It occurs after lymph vessels or lymph nodes are removed or treated with radiation.

Malignant—Cancerous, describes cells with a tendency to spread to other organs.

Margin—Edge or border of the tissue removed in cancer surgery.

"Clean margin" / "negative margin"—Terms used when

a pathologist finds no cancer cells at the edge of the tissue, suggesting that all of the cancer has been removed.

"Positive" / "involved margin"—Terms used when a pathologist finds cancer cells at the edge of the tissue, suggesting that all of the cancer has not been removed.

Metastatic—Describes cancers that spread via the blood or lymphatic system to other parts of the body to form secondary tumors.

Millimeter—Measure of length in the metric system often used to measure tumors. There are 25 millimeters to 1 inch.

Mucositis—Complication of some cancer therapies in which the lining of the digestive system becomes inflamed. It is often seen as sores in the mouth.

Negative test result—Test result that does not indicate the specific disease or condition for which the test was being done.

Neoplasm—Another word for tumor.

Neuropathy—Condition that causes numbness, tingling, burning, or weakness. It usually begins in the hands or foot and can be caused by certain anticancer drugs.

Neutropenia—Abnormal decrease in the number of neutropils, a type of white blood cell.

Patient advocate—Person who helps a patient work with others who have an effect on the patient's health, including doctors, insurance companies, employers, case managers, and lawyers. A patient advocate helps resolve issues about health care, medical bills, and job discrimination related to a patient's medical condition.

Port—Implanted device through which blood may be withdrawn and drugs may be infused without repeated needle sticks.

Port-a-cath—Another term for a port.

Positive test result—Test result that reveals the presence of a specific disease or condition for which the test is being done.

Primary tumor—Place where the cancer first started to grow.

Protocol—Outline or action plan for a treatment program.

Radiation therapy—Use of high-energy radiation from X-rays, neutrons, and other sources to kill cancer cells and shrink tumors. Also called radiotherapy.

Radical mastectomy—Surgery for breast cancer in which the breast, chest muscles, and all of the lymph nodes under the arm are removed. Doctors consider radical mastectomy only when the tumor has spread to the chest muscles.

Refractory cancer—Cancer that does not respond to treatment. Also called resistant cancer.

Regimen—Treatment plan that specifies the dosage, schedule, and duration of treatment.

Regional—In oncology, describes the body area right around a tumor.

Regression—Decrease in the size of a tumor or in the extent of cancer in the body.

Remission—Decrease or disappearance of signs and symptoms of cancer.

Resected—Removed by surgery.

Resistant cancer—Another term for refractory cancer.

Response rate—Percentage of patients whose cancer shrinks or disappears after treatment.

Second-line therapy—Treatment given when initial treatment doesn't work or stops working.

Sentinel lymph node—First lymph node to which cancer is likely to spread from the primary tumor. When cancer spreads, the cancer cells may appear first in the sentinel node before spreading to other lymph nodes.

Stage—Extent of a cancer in the body. Staging is usually based on the size of a tumor, whether lymph nodes contain cancer, and whether the cancer has spread from the original site to other parts of the body. There are four stages: Stage I is localized, small, and easily treatable. Stages II and III are incrementally further developed. Stage IV cancer has spread to other organs with surgery no longer being an option.

Staging—Performing exams and tests to learn the extent of the cancer within the body, especially whether it has spread from the original site to other parts of the body.

T cell—Type of white blood cell that attacks virus-infected cells, foreign cells, and cancer cells. T cells also produce a number of substances that regulate the immune response.

Tumor—Abnormal mass of tissue that results when cells divide more than they should or do not die when they should. Tumors may be benign or malignant.

Tumor marker—Proteins and other substances in the blood that indicate the presence of cancer cells somewhere else in the body.

White blood cells—General term for the cells in the body that play a major role in battling infection.

resources

Services That Provide Help Along the Way

There are scores of terrific nonprofit organizations whose sole purpose is to provide a huge array of amazingly generous, useful, free services to people with cancer and their families. Here are a few extraordinary ones.

PATIENT ADVOCATE FOUNDATION
(www.patientadvocate.org; 800-532-5274)
National nonprofit organization that works as a liaison between patients and employers, insurers, and creditors to resolve insurance, job discrimination, and/or debt crisis matters relative to their diagnosis. Its state-by-state financial resource guide lets you locate assistance for seeking relief from many illness-related expenses, from medication to food and utilities.

AMERICAN CANCER SOCIETY
(www.cancer.org; 800-ACS-2345)

Hope Lodge Free, temporary housing facilities for cancer patients undergoing treatment. Homelike nurturing environment, run by ACS. Twenty-two lodges currently exist.

Look Good, Feel Better Volunteer beauty professionals lead small groups and give techniques for skin care, nail care, makeup techniques, and options related to hair loss. (For free step-by-step guides and tips, call 800-395-5665.)

ACS will also lend you a wig or hairpiece if you choose not to buy one. This is a good way to test out wearing a wig before you buy one. Another possible lending source is the social work department at the hospital where you're being treated.

LIVESTRONG (The Lance Armstrong Foundation: www.livestrong.org; 866-235-7205)
Survivorship Notebook, the best free resource I've found, and it's free except for $10 shipping and handling. Get it. It'll help you immensely.

CANCER SURVIVAL BOX
(www.cancersurvivalbox.org)
Six-CD set that provides information and resources regarding most types of cancer.

CANCER HOPE NETWORK
(www.cancerhopenetwork.org)
Confidential one-on-one support for survivors and families. You are matched with a trained volunteer who has recovered from a similar cancer and is of a similar age, living arrangement, or other general circumstances.

CARINGBRIDGE (www.caringbridge.org)
Provides free, easy-to-create personalized Web sites. You can keep friends and family informed and they can visit and leave messages. Available in all fifty states.

THE WELLNESS COMMUNITY
(www.thewellnesscommunity.org)
Wonderful online support groups, nutrition information, mind/body exercises, and education.

Y-ME NATIONAL BREAST CANCER ORGANIZATION
(www.y-me.org; 800-221-2141 for English
language and interpreters in 150 languages,
800-986-9505 for Spanish language)
Breast cancer twenty-four-hour hotline that's free and confidential. Trained peer counselors are breast cancer survivors who will answer questions and match you with a survivor who had a similar diagnosis or life experience.

Magazines

Coping With Cancer (www.copingmag.com;
615-791-3859) $19 for 6 issues per year
P.O. Box 682268, Franklin, TN 37068–2268
Cure (www.curetoday.com) Free subscription.

Retreats

Camp Mak-A-Dream (www.campdream.org;
406-549-5987)
Free camp for cancer patients ages six to twenty-five; charge for adults over twenty-five. Located in Missoula, Montana. Open all year.

First Descents (www.firstdescents.org; 970-476-9400)
Free summer camp in Vail, Colorado, for young adults over age eighteen. Kayaking, horseback riding, rock climbing, fishing.

Life Beyond Cancer (www.lifebeyondcancer.org)
For women cancer survivors. Free four-day retreat in Tucson, Arizona, held every December.

Stowe Weekend of Hope (www.stowehope.org;
800-GO-STOWE)

Located in Stowe, Vermont. Held each spring for cancer survivors and their families. Free accommodations for first-time guests. Most events are free.

Commonweal Cancer Help Program (www.commonweal.org; 415-868-0814)
One-week retreats held three times every spring and fall. Several locations in the U.S. and Canada. Fees are approximately $2,000 per person.

Mail-order Resources

The Cancer Club Store (www.cancerclub.com; 800-586-9062)
Gifts and inspiration for people dealing with cancer.

Choose Hope (www.choosehope.com; 888-348-4673)
Terrific catalog offering cancer-related items from apparel (including my personal favorite: "CANCER SUCKS" T-shirts, caps, and pins), to jewelry, caps, and even a "Cancer Daze" chemo care package and a Radiation Skin Care Bag. It also offers "queasy drops" hard candies. Started by a cancer survivor, this company donates 10–20 percent of its gross sales to cancer research and service organizations, which it lists on its Web site.

As you can see, I'm a big fan of this organization. The Web site also offers links to support organizations and other helpful information.

"tlc" Tender Loving Care catalog

(www.tlccatalog.org; 800-850-9445)

Offered by the American Cancer Society, wigs and related items are extremely inexpensive. Prices are the best I've found anywhere.

CDC Division of Cancer Prevention and Control's List of Best Overall Cancer Web Sites

The following organizations are affiliated with the Center for Disease Control's Division of Cancer Prevention and Control, and their Web sites offer the highest-caliber help and information:

American Cancer Society: www.cancer.org; 800-ACS-2345

Avon Foundation Breast Care Fund: www.avon breastcare.org; 212-695-3081

Cancer*Care:* www.cancercare.org; 800-813-4673

Children's Oncology Camp Foundation/Camp Mak-A-Dream: www.campdream.org; 406-549-5987

Dana Farber Cancer Institute: www.dfci.harvard.edu; 866-408-3324

Gilda's Club Worldwide: www.gildasclub.org; 888-445-3248

The Lance Armstrong Foundation: www.livestrong. org; 866-235-7205

M. D. Anderson Cancer Center: www.mdanderson. org; 800-392-1611

Men Against Breast Cancer: www.menagainstbreast cancer.org; 866-547-6222

The National Coalition for Cancer Survivorship: www.canceradvocacy.org; 877-622-7937

Patient Advocate Foundation: www.patient advocate.org; 800-532-5274

The Susan G. Komen Breast Cancer Foundation: www.komen.org; 800-462-9273

Cancer Awareness Colors

All cancers: Lavender
Bladder: Yellow
Brain: Gray
Breast: Pink
Cervical: White
Childhood: Gold
Colon: Dark Blue

Esophageal: Periwinkle

Head and neck: Burgundy

Kidney: Kelly green

Leiposarcoma: Purple

Leukemia: Orange

Liver: Emerald

Lung: Pearl

Lymphoma: Lime

Melanoma: Black

Multiple myaloma: Burgundy

Ovarian: Teal

Pancreatic: Purple

Prostate: Light blue

Sarcoma / Bone: Yellow

Uterine: Peach

for further reading

Top Ten Cancer Books

IT'S NOT ABOUT THE BIKE: My Journey Back to Life,
Lance Armstrong and Sally Jenkins
World athlete Lance Armstrong attests that the fight
against cancer makes even the Tour de France look
easy. But moreover, he declares that his battle showed
him what true beauty really is and where life's priorities
belong. Read this book. It encourages with grace and
honesty without diminishing the challenges of getting
through cancer.

BREAST CANCER HUSBAND: How to Help Your Wife
(and Yourself) Through Diagnosis, Treatment and Beyond,
Marc Silver
This book provides great insight into men's responses
to illness and gives wonderful guidance to husbands
on how to provide support to their wives, including

specific instructions on how to discuss concerns, ask questions, and listen productively. Full of valuable, practical information.

WHEN IT'S CANCER: The 10 Essential Steps to Follow After Your Diagnosis, Toni Bernay and Saar Porath
Co-written by a world renowned pioneering breast oncologist who was diagnosed with cancer, and his wife, a preeminient psychologist, this book provides a program for taking control of cancer before it takes control of your life. Emotional, logistical, and medical strategies for remaining proactive as you navigate your way through cancer treatment are all covered.

GETTING WELL AGAIN, O. Carl Simonton, M.D., Stephanie Matthews-Simonton, and James Creighton
This classic walks you through the fear, confusion, and questions that accompany cancer and provides exercises and information to help you cope with and manage difficult issues in a positive manner.

EVERY SECOND COUNTS, Lance Armstrong
Armstrong confronts the issue of moving beyond life with cancer and applies the insights he gained through his illness to subsequent challenges.

CANCER VIXEN: A TRUE STORY,
Marisa Acocella Marchetto

Everyone I know who has read this (including me) will tell you that once you pick up this book, which is done in a cartoon format, you can't put it down. It's written and illustrated by a successful Manhattan cartoonist fashionista who's engaged to a hot New York City restaurateur when she learns she has breast cancer. A big soul, lots of courage, great friends, and an amazing, irreverent sense of humor get her through.

WHY I WORE LIPSTICK TO MY MASTECTOMY,
Geralyn Lucas

Another charming memoir that proves that humor is a major part of overcoming the horrors of cancer. The author shares her struggles with her sense of sexuality and self-image, and what she learned on her own when she couldn't find guidance on how to cope.

LOVE, MEDICINE AND MIRACLES, Bernie Siegel, M.D.
A positive reminder that attitude plays a large role in moving through illness to health.

HAPPINESS IN A STORM: Facing Illness and Embracing Life as a Healthy Survivor,
Wendy Schlessel Harpham

A physician and three-time cancer survivor shares the guidelines she has developed for getting through cancer. A sensible, realistic guide that illustrates how to cope with the fallout from serious illness and still nourish joy.

SAVING GRACES: Finding Solace and Strength from Friends and Strangers, Elizabeth Edwards

Elizabeth Edwards's diagnosis of breast cancer was the second major blow in her life. The first was the death of her teenage son. This book is about the sustenance and importance of community and the support of others when we face a tragedy that seems too hard to bear.

Breast Cancer

DR. SUSAN LOVE'S BREAST BOOK, Fourth Edition,
Dr. Susan Love and Karen Lindsey

Dr. Susan Love is cofounder of the National Breast Cancer Coalition and associate professor of clinical surgery at UCLA School of Medicine. This is the bible of breast cancer books. Although it deals with all areas of breast health, it provides a comprehensive discussion of the latest research and recommendations for breast care and cancer treatment.

LIVING BEYOND BREAST CANCER—A Survivor's Guide for When Treatment Ends and the Rest of Your Life Begins, Marissa C. Weiss, M.D., and Ellen Weiss
Written by a radiation oncologist, this book provides a guide for returning to "normal life" after breast cancer. It covers everything from pain control, weight management, and hormone and tamoxifen therapy to alternative treatments and navigating the emotional terrain of fears and uncertainties. Endorsed by Bernie Siegel and former surgeon general C. Everett Koop.

A BREAST CANCER JOURNEY: Your Personal Guidebook, Second Edition, American Cancer Society
This book includes information about treatment options, the latest surgical techniques for breast reconstruction, drug therapies, complementary and alternative methods, detailed questions to ask your medical team, and wellness plans for recovery and life after cancer.

Childhood Cancers

LIVING WITH CHILDHOOD CANCER: A Practical Guide to Help Families Cope, Leigh A. Woznick and Carol D. Goodheart, American Psychological Association
Anna T. Meadows, MD, a senior oncologist at the Children's Hospital of Philadelphia, calls this book "an excellent roadmap for families . . . faced with the shattering experience of having a child with cancer." Includes chapters on pain relief, side effects, fostering a child's psychological development, nurturing your child's self-esteem and a large resource section of organizations, support groups, Web sites, books, and videos.

Children's Books

BECKY AND THE WORRY CUP, Wendy S. Harpham, see also *When a Parent Has Cancer*

OUR MOM HAS CANCER, Abigail and Adrienne Ackerman, American Cancer Society
Two sisters, ages nine and eleven, describe what it was like for them when their mother was diagnosed with cancer. It is an honest, hopeful account of the year that

their mother underwent surgery and chemotherapy written in a relatable style for kids.

OUR FAMILY HAS CANCER, TOO!
Christine Clifford
Provides the knowledge that "you're not alone," information about cancer, and a place for children to write down questions for parents, doctors, and teachers and draw pictures that represent their feelings for later discussion. Ages seven to twelve.

BECAUSE SOMEONE I LOVE HAS CANCER
Kid's Activity Book, American Cancer Society
Support, encouragement, and information for children ages six to twelve. Creative activities allow your child to work through unfamiliar feelings and learn to recognize and tap into positive moments.

Complementary and Alternative Medicines

The books in this section have all been recommended by the Cancer Patient Education Network of the National Cancer Institute

CHOICES IN HEALING: Integrating the Best of Conventional and Complementary Approaches to Cancer, Michael Lerner

Contains thorough discussions and evaluations of complementary programs—spiritual, psychological, nutritional, and pharmaceutical—as well as other less conventional approaches. Although the author believes that all people with cancer should be under the care of an oncologist, he provides a wealth of information that helps to clarify the overwhelming amount of data on alternative treatments.

AMERICAN CANCER SOCIETY'S GUIDE TO COMPLEMENTARY AND ALTERNATIVE CANCER METHODS, Second Edition, American Cancer Society

The ACS reminds us that not all nontraditional methods of treating cancer are created equally. This is an up-to-date comprehensive volume with expert contributors who examine the evidence, both pro and con, for more than two hundred treatment methods.

General

AMERICAN CANCER SOCIETY CONSUMER GUIDE TO CANCER DRUGS, Second Edition, Gail Wilkes

Explains cancer drugs to nonprofessionals and lists side effects and precautions for more than two hundred cancer-related medicines.

*AMERICAN CANCER SOCIETY'S GUIDE TO PAIN
CONTROL: Understanding and Managing Cancer
Pain, Revised Edition,* **American Cancer Society**
There are lots of pain relief options, and there's no reason for you to live with unnecessary pain. Simple, invaluable information on how to work with your health care team to create a plan that balances pain relief and the potential side effects of pain medications.

*WHEN A PARENT HAS CANCER: A Guide for
Caring for Your Children,* **Wendy S. Harpham**
The author—a mother, physician, and cancer survivor—draws on all of her experiences to teach parents how to help their children cope with the fears and life-changing demands that cancer places on everyone in the family. Includes an illustrated children's story, *Becky and the Worry Cup,* that illustrates the concerns kids have and ways to address them.

Ovarian Cancer

*GILDA'S DISEASE: Sharing Personal Experiences
and a Medical Perspective on Ovarian Cancer,*
Steven Piver, M.D.
Piver, the chief of gynecological oncology at Roswell Park Cancer Institute, collaborated with Gene Wilder (the husband of Gilda Radner, for whom the book is

named) to provide more information on ovarian cancer for women. The book outlines medical treatments and alternative therapies.

Prostate Cancer

DR. PATRICK WALSH'S GUIDE TO SURVIVING PROSTATE CANCER, Second Edition, Patrick C. Walsh, M.D. and Janet Farrar Worthington
Recommended by the Prostate Cancer Foundation and generally agreed to be the best book on prostate cancer. Explains the newest treatment options available and important lifestyle factors for longterm health.

PROSTATE CANCER FOR DUMMIES, Paul H. Lange, M.D. and Christine Adamec
Recommended by the Prostate Cancer Foundation, this book provides straightforward information on treatment options, coping with side effects, and handling the demands of daily life and necessary follow-up care.

puzzle solution

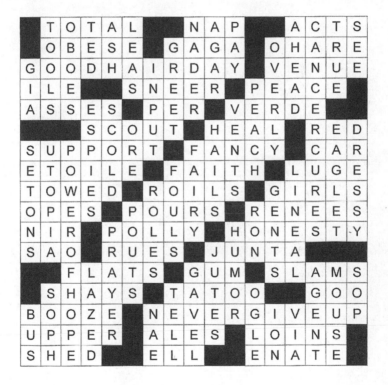

acknowledgments

It must take more than a village to raise a child, because it takes a small cosmos to raise a book. This one is the result of great generosity of spirit on the part of those who have gone through cancer treatment and shared their hard won knowledge so that others' journeys might be eased. My thanks to them appears in the front of this book on pages vii and viii. My special thanks and great admiration go to Abbie Wood, the first to share her wisdom with me to ease my own cancer journey. She is the reason this book exists.

Anything you do is easier when you have a group of friends supporting your effort, and many friends have been an amazing encouragement and support to me. My deepest thanks go to Rich Barber, who encouraged me to take a risk, Joe Barnett, Hannah Bekritsky, Therese Borchard, ace photographer Richard Corson and Connie Corson, Andrea Doering, Anthony DeStefano, Kimberly DeStefano, Lauren Gorman, John Greenman, Jerry Horn, Adrienne Ingrum, Carol Johnson, Joan and

Bob Kowal, Liz Leahey, Grace Maher, Jonathan, Francie and Lucy Miller, Nancy S. Pines, Jerry and Jeannie Schieb, Susanna Schindler, Barbara Sheri, Lucia Staniels Tasker, Betsy Wilson, the Wood family: Rebecca, Lance, Summer, Lance Lee and Brady, and my friends at Church-in-the-Gardens.

Everybody should have physicians as accomplished, dedicated, intelligent, and caring as Dr. David Berman and Dr. Avram Abramowitz. They are my angels.

Special thanks go to the authors of the original cancer prayers in this book: Rabbi Nathan Goldberg, Imam Yusuf Hasan, and Reverend Noel Vanek, as well as to Christine Clifford Beckwith for providing the cartoons that appear throughout.

I've seen Rolf Zettersten direct on Broadway, and he's also a maestro when it comes to publishing. Of course, it helps that he has an extraordinary team. My special thanks to him and to Chris Park, my editor, who is great at what she does and makes it look much easier than it is; to Sarah Sper, who clearly has a great future in publishing; art director Jody Waldrup; Tareth Mitch, production editor extraordinaire; and the rest of the Center Street team.

Finally, my thanks and love to my husband Bob, who is my biggest fan and my present from God. He saw me through my own days without hair, and from the look in his eyes you'd have thought he was looking at Miss America.

index

About the Author

B.C. (before cancer), Michelle Rapkin would have told you about her work. Now, however, she knows better. She is a wife, sister, friend, step-mother and grandmother, and she lives with her husband in Forest Hills, New York.

Dear Reader:

If you have any of your own hints, tips, information, or tools that you would like to share with others who are fighting cancer, please send them, along with your name and contact information, to mrapkin@peoplepc.com.